CLINICAL DECISION
MANUAL

COMPANION TO
KELLEY'S TEXTBOOK
OF INTERNAL MEDICINE

Fourth Edition

CLINICAL DECISION MANUAL

COMPANION TO
KELLEY'S TEXTBOOK
OF INTERNAL MEDICINE
Fourth Edition

Edited by
Kim A. Eagle, MD
Chief of Clinical Cardiology
Co-Director Heart Care Program
Senior Associate Chair,
Department of Internal Medicine
University of Michigan Medical Center
Ann Arbor, Michigan

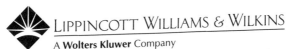

LIPPINCOTT WILLIAMS & WILKINS
A **Wolters Kluwer** Company
Philadelphia · Baltimore · New York · London
Buenos Aires · Hong Kong · Sydney · Tokyo

Acquisitions Editor: Richard Winters
Developmental Editor: Sarah Kane
Production Editor: Patrick Carr
Manufacturing Manager: Benjamin Rivera
Cover Designer: QT Design
Cover Logo Designer: Jeane Norton
Compositor: Maryland Composition
Printer: P. R. Donnelley, Crawfordsville

© 2001 by LIPPINCOTT WILLIAMS & WILKINS
530 Walnut Street
Philadelphia, PA 19106 USA
LWW.com

Printed in the USA

Library of Congress Cataloging-in-Publication Data

Clinical decision manual: for use with the 4th edition of Kelley's textbook of internal medicine/edited by Kim A. Eagle.
    p.; cm.
Includes bibliographical references and index.
ISBN 0-7817-2222-5
    1. Medical protocols. 2. Clinical medicine—Decision making. 3. Evidence-based medicine. I. Eagle, Kim A. II. Kelley's textbook of internal medicine, 4th ed.
    [DNLM: 1. Internal Medicine—methods—Handbooks. 2. Decision Making—Handbooks. WB 115 K29 2000 Suppl. 2000]
RC64.C54 2000
616—dc21

00-061844

10 9 8 7 6 5 4 3 2 1

DEDICATION

To Darlene and Taylor . . . for their unending encourage-
ment and support.

CONTENTS

xi

PREFACE

The Clinical Decision Manual has been developed for use by busy clinicians. With the ever-increasing pace of medicine and the amount of knowledge expanding continuously, busy practitioners are looking for simple methods for allowing rapid access to evidence-based tools that help in the evaluation and/or management of common conditions. This compendium of algorithms, tables, and figures is designed to help clinicians right at the bedside, as they wrestle with a variety of clinical problems.

The Clinical Decision Guides have been selected from literally scores of decision algorithms and tables included in the fourth edition of *Kelley's Textbook of Internal Medicine*. Each guide has been graded based on the level of scientific evidence, giving the user an appropriate level of confidence surrounding the scientific information provided. Tables and figures that are labeled **Evidence Level: A** are based upon national guidelines or highly robust clinical trials. **Evidence Level: B** refers to material based upon a limited amount of trial information or large observational studies. **Evidence Level: C** decision aids are based primarily upon expert consensus. The category indication appears just below the legend or caption of each figure or table.

The Clinical Decision Guides are intended for use in the daily care of patients. I believe that providers will find this information to be very useful in real time as they create the most appropriate and evidenced-based care possible for patients with common conditions.

Kim A. Eagle, MD

CLINICAL DECISION MANUAL

COMPANION TO
KELLEY'S TEXTBOOK
OF INTERNAL MEDICINE

Fourth Edition

1

CARDIOLOGY

TABLE 1.1. PRIMARY PREVENTION OF CARDIOVASCULAR DISEASES

Risk Intervention	Recommendations
Smoking Goal: complete cessation	Ask about smoking status as part of routine evaluation. Reinforce nonsmoking status. Strongly encourage patients and family to stop smoking. Provide counseling, nicotine replacement, and formal cessation programs as appropriate.
Blood pressure control Goal: <140/90 mm Hg or <130/85 mm Hg if heart failure, renal insufficiency, or diabetes	Measure blood pressure in all adults at least every 2 yr. Promote lifestyle modification: weight control, physical activity, moderation in alcohol intake, and moderate sodium restriction. If blood pressure ≥140/90 mm Hg after 6 months of lifestyle modification, or if initial blood pressure >160/100 mm Hg or >130/85 mm Hg with heart failure, renal insufficiency, or diabetes, add blood pressure medication. Individualize therapy to patient's age, race, need for drugs with specific benefits, etc.
Cholesterol management Primary goal: LDL <160 mg/dL if 0–1 risk factors or LDL <130 mg/dL if ≥2 risk factors Secondary goals: HDL >35 mg/dL, TG <200 mg/dL	Ask about dietary habits as part of routine evaluation. Measure total and HDL cholesterol in all adults ≥20 yr old and assess positive and negative risk factors at least every 5 yr. For all persons: promote American Heart Association Step 1 diet (≤30% fat, <10% saturated fat, <300 mg/d cholesterol), weight control, and physical activity. Measure LDL if total cholesterol ≥240 mg/dL or ≥200 mg/dL with ≥2 risk factors or if HDL <35 mg/dL. If LDL ≥160 mg/dL with 0–1 risk factors or ≥130 mg/dL on 2 occasions with ≥2 risk factors, then Start Step II diet (≤30% fat, <7% saturated fat, <200 mg/dL cholesterol) and weight control. Rule out secondary causes of high LDL (LFTs, TFTs, UA). If LDL ≥160 mg/dL plus 2 risk factors or ≥190 mg/dL or	Risk factors: age (men ≥45 yr, women ≥55 yr or postmenopausal), hypertension, diabetes, smoking, HDL <35 mg/dL, family history of CHD in first-degree relatives (in male relatives <55 yr, female relatives <65 yr) HDL ≥60 mg/dL, subtract 1 risk factor from the number of positive risk factors.

≥220 mg/dL in men <35 yr old or in premenopausal women, then consider adding drug therapy to diet therapy for LDL levels >those listed above that persist despite Step II diet.

Suggested drug therapy for high LDL levels (≥160 mg/dL) (drug selection priority modified according to TG level)

TG <200 mg/dL	TG 200–400 mg/dL	Tg >400 mg/dL	HDL <35 mg/dL: Emphasize weight
Statin	Statin	Consider combined	management and physical activity,
Resin	Niacin	drug therapy	avoidance of cigarette smoking.
Niacin		(niacin, fibrates, statin)	Niacin raises HDL. Consider niacin if patient has ≥2 risk factors and high LDL (except patients with diabetes).

Physical activity
Goal: Exercise regularly 3–4 times per week for 30–60 min

Weight management
Goal: BMI 21–25 kg/m²

Diabetes management
Near normal fasting plasma glucose and near normal HbA1c (<7)

Estrogens

If LDL goal not achieved, consider combination drug therapy.
Ask about physical activity status and exercise habits as part of routine evaluation.
Encourage 30 min of vigorous dynamic exercise 3–4 times per week as well as increased physical activity in daily lifestyle activities (e.g., walking breaks at work, gardening, household work).
Advise medically supervised programs for those with low functional capacity and/or comorbid conditions.
Measure patient's weight and height. BMI, and waist-to-hip ratio at each visit as part of routine evaluation.
Start weight management and physical activity as appropriate. Desirable BMI range: 21–25 kg/m².
Desirable waist circumference <40 inches in men and <36 inches in women.
Appropriate hypoglycemic therapy to achieve near-normal fasting plasma glucose as indicated by HbA1c.
Treatment of other risks (e.g., physical activity, weight management, and blood pressure; for cholesterol management, see recommendations for patients with coronary disease in Table 1.29.4.

Consider estrogen replacement in all postmenopausal women, especially those with multiple CHD risk factors.
Individualize recommendation according to other health risks.

TG, triglycerides; LFTs, liver function tests; TFTs, thyroid function tests; UA, uric acid; CHD, coronary heart disease; BMI, body mass index (704.5); HDL, high-density lipoprotein; LDL, low-density lipoprotein.

EVIDENCE LEVEL: A. Reference: Consensus Panel Statement. Guide to primary prevention of cardiovascular diseases. *Circulation* 1997;95:2330.

Management of Hypercholesterolemia in High-Risk Primary Prevention of ASCVD

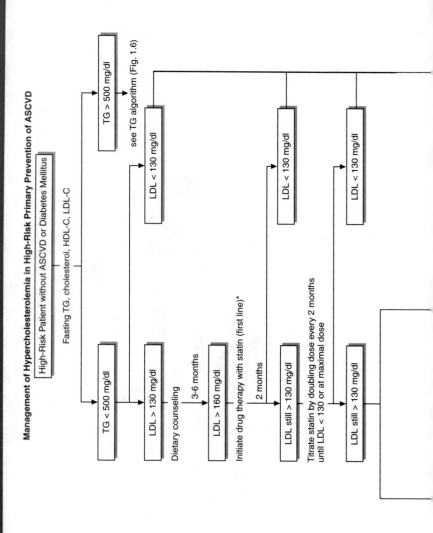

High-Risk Patient without ASCVD or Diabetes Mellitus

Fasting TG, cholesterol, HDL-C, LDL-C

TG < 500 mg/dl

TG > 500 mg/dl

see TG algorithm (Fig. 1.6)

LDL > 130 mg/dl

LDL < 130 mg/dl

Dietary counseling

3-6 months

LDL > 160 mg/dl

Initiate drug therapy with statin (first line)*

2 months

LDL still > 130 mg/dl

LDL < 130 mg/dl

Titrate statin by doubling dose every 2 months
until LDL < 130 or at maximal dose

LDL still > 130 mg/dl

LDL < 130 mg/dl

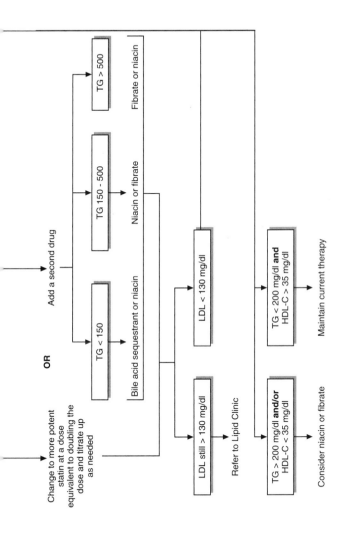

Change to more potent
statin at a dose
equivalent to doubling the
dose and titrate up
as needed

OR

Add a second drug

| TG < 150 | TG 150 - 500 | TG > 500 |

Bile acid sequestrant or niacin

Niacin or fibrate

Fibrate or niacin

LDL still > 130 mg/dl

Refer to Lipid Clinic

LDL < 130 mg/dl

TG > 200 mg/dl **and/or**
HDL-C < 35 mg/dl

Consider niacin or fibrate

TG < 200 mg/dl **and**
HDL-C > 35 mg/dl

Maintain current therapy

* Niacin or bile acid sequestrants could be considered instead

FIGURE 1.2. Strategy for the management of hypercholesterolemia in the primary prevention of CHD in patients with two or more risk factors for CHD.
EVIDENCE LEVEL: C. Expert Opinion.

MANAGEMENT OF HYPERCHOLESTEROLEMIA IN HIGH-RISK PRIMARY PREVENTION OF ASCVD

5

TABLE 1.3. COMPREHENSIVE RISK REDUCTION FOR PATIENTS WITH CORONARY AND OTHER VASCULAR DISEASE

Risk Intervention	Recommendations
Smoking Goal: complete cessation	Strongly encourage patient and family to stop smoking. Provide counseling, nicotine replacement, and formal cessation programs as appropriate.
BP control Goal: <140/90 mm Hg or <130/85 mm Hg if heart failure, renal insufficiency, or diabetes	Initiate lifestyle modification—weight control, physical activity, moderation in alcohol intake, and moderate sodium restriction in all patients with blood pressure ≥130 mm Hg systolic or 85 mm Hg diastolic. Add blood pressure medication, individualized to other patient requirements and characteristics (i.e., age, race, need for drugs with specific benefits) if blood pressure is not <140 mm Hg systolic or 90 mm Hg diastolic or if blood pressure is not <130 mm Hg systolic or <85 mm Hg diastolic for individuals with heart failure, renal insufficiency, or diabetes.
Lipid management Primary goal: LDL <100 mg/dL Secondary goals: HDL >35 mg/dL, TG <200 mg/dL	Start American Heart Association Step II diet in all patients (≤30% fat, <7% saturated fat, <200 mg/d cholesterol) and promote physical activity. Assess fasting lipid profile. In post-MI patients, lipid profile may take 4 to 6 weeks to stabilize. Add drug therapy according to the following guide.

LDL <100 md/dL	LDL 100–130 mg/dL	LDL >130 mg/dL	HDL <35 mg/dL
No drug therapy	Consider drug therapy to diet, as follows	Add drug therapy to diet, as follows	Emphasize weight management and physical activity. Advise smoking cessation. If needed to achieve LDL goals, consider niacin, statin, fibrates.
	⎰Suggested drug therapy⎱		
	TG <200 mg/dL	TG 200–400 mg/dL	TG >400 mg/dL
	Statin Resin Niacin	Statin Niacin	Consider combined drug therapy (niacin, fibrates, statin)
	If LDL goal not achieved, consider combination drug therapy.		

Physical activity Minimum goal: 30 min 3 to 4 times per week	Assess risk, preferably with exercise test, to guide prescription. Encourage minimum of 30–60 min of activity 3–4 times weekly (walking, jogging, cycling, or other aerobic activity) supplemented by an increase in daily lifestyle activities (e.g., walking breaks at work, gardening, household work). Maximun benefit 5 to 6 hours a week. Advise medically supervised programs for moderate- to high-risk patients.
Weight management Goal: BMI 21–25 kg/m²	Measure patient's weight and height, BMI, and waist-to-hip ratio at each visit as part of routine evaluation. Start weight management and physical activity as appropriate. Desirable BMI range: 21–25 kg/m². Desirable waist circumference <40 inches in men and <36 increase in women.
Diabetes management Near normal fasting plasma glucose and near normal HbA1c (<7)	Appropriate hypoglycemic therapy to achieve near-normal fasting plasma glucose as indicated by HbA1c. Treatment of other risks (e.g., physical activity, weight management, and blood pressure; for cholesterol management see earlier recommendations).
Antiplatelet agents/anticoagulants	Start aspirin 80–325 mg/d if not contraindicated. Manage warfarin to international normalized ratio = 2–3.5 post-MI patients not able to take aspirin.
ACE inhibitors post-MI	Start early post-MI in stable high-risk patients (anterior MI, previous MI, Killip class II [S₃ gallop, rates, radiographic CHF]). Continue indefinitely for all with LV dysfunction (ejection fraction ≤40%) or symptoms of failure. Use as needed to manage blood pressure or symptoms in all other patients.
β-blockers	Start in high-risk post-MI patients (arrhythmia, LV dysfunction, inducible ischemia) at 5–28 days. Continue 6 mo minimum. Observe usual contraindications. Use as needed to manage angina, rhythm, or blood pressure in all other patients.
Estrogens	Estrogen replacement: individualize according to other health risks.

BP, blood pressure; BMI, body mass index; HbA1c;, LD, low-density lipoprotein; HDL, high-density lipoprotein; MI, myocardial infarction; TG, triglycerides; ACE, angiotensin-converting enzyme.

EVIDENCE LEVEL: A. Reference: Consensus Panel Statement. Preventing heart atttack and death in patients with coronary disease. *Circulation* 1995;92:2–4.

COMPREHENSIVE RISK REDUCTION FOR PATIENTS WITH CORONARY AND OTHER VASCULAR DISEASE

Management of Hypercholesterolemia in Patients with ASCVD or Diabetes Mellitus

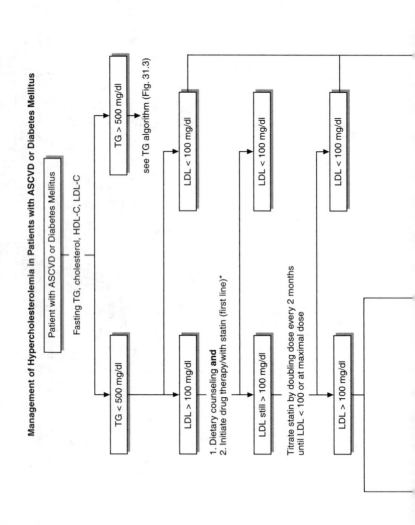

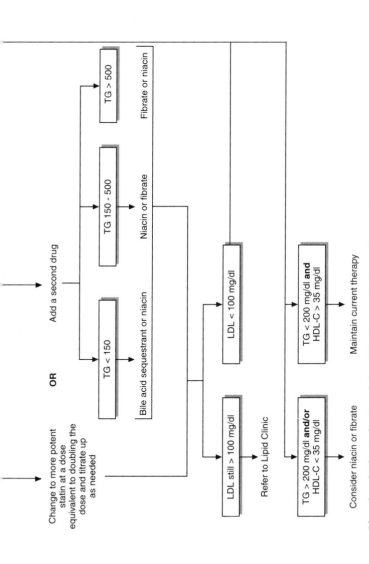

FIGURE 1.4. Strategy for the management of hypercholesterolemia in the secondary prevention of CHD in patients with established CHD.
EVIDENCE LEVEL: **C. Expert Opinion.**

MANAGEMENT OF HYPERCHOLESTEROLEMIA IN PATIENTS WITH ASCVD OR DIABETES MELLITUS

9

Treatment of Hypercholesterolemia

No CHD or Other Atherosclerotic Disease

Measuring non-fasting total cholesterol and HDL-C
Assess Risk Factors (RF)
- Age: Male ≥ 45 years; Female ≥ 55 years or postmenopausal w/o estrogen replacement tx
- Family h/o premature CHD: Male MI < 55 years; Female MI < 65 years
- HDL-C < 35 mg/dl
- Hypertension
- Current smoker
- Diabetes
- Positive RF:HDL-C ≥ 60 (subtract one RF from analysis)

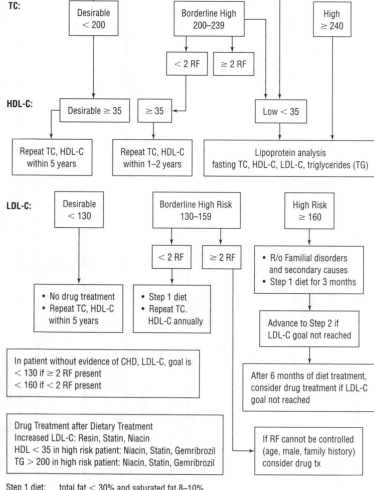

Step 1 diet: total fat < 30% and saturated fat 8–10%
of total calories < 300mg cholesterol per day
Step 2 diet: total fat < 30% and saturated fat < 7% of total calories; < 200mg cholesterol per day

EVIDENCE LEVEL: A. Reference: Expert panel on detection, evaluation and treatment of high blood cholesterol in adults. Summary of the second report of the National Cholesterol Education Program Expert Panel (Adult Treatment Panel II). JAMA 1993; 269: 3015–23

CARDIOLOGY

CHD or Other Atherosclerotic Disease*

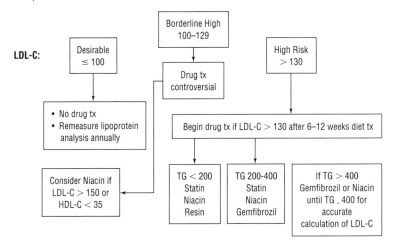

Measure fasting lipoprotein analysis
- R/o familial disorders and secondary causes of abnormal lipids
- Step 2 diet

In patient with CHD, goal LDL-C is ≤ 100
Secondary goals: HDL-C ≥ 35 and TG < 200

LDL-C:

Desirable
≤ 100

Borderline High
100–129

High Risk
> 130

Drug tx
controversial

- No drug tx
- Remeasure lipoprotein analysis annually

Begin drug tx if LDL-C > 130 after 6–12 weeks diet tx

Consider Niacin if
LDL-C > 150 or
HDL-C < 35

TG < 200
Statin
Niacin
Resin

TG 200-400
Statin
Niacin
Gemfibrozil

If TG > 400
Gemfibrozil or Niacin
until TG , 400 for
accurate
calculation of LDL-C

Medication	Dosage	Side Effects	Caution
Statins	Pravastatin 10–40mg QD Lovastatin 10–80mg QD Fluvastatin 20–40mg QD Simvastatin 5–80mg QD Atorvastatin 10–80mg QD	Myopathy, hepatitis Monitor LFT's	Use with caution in combination with gemfibrozil, niacin, cyclosporin, erythromycin
Niacin	1.5–6gm QD (BID or TID) start at 250mg BID and titrate up	Flushing, hepatitis Monitor LFT's, glucose, uric acid	Contraindicated in PUD, liver disease, gout, diabetes, hepatoxicity is dose related
Resins	Cholestyramine 4–12mg BID Colestipol 5–15mg BID	Increase TG, GI distress	Do not use in patients with increased TG. Associated with decreased absorption of some drugs
Gemfibrozil	600mg BID	GI distress Cholelithiasis Myopathy Follow LFT's	Contraindicated in renal failure Lower dose in renal insufficiency Follow PT when on warfarin

*Atherosclerotic disease including
thrombotic stroke, carotid disease,
claudication, arterial bruit

Special caution with combined drug treatment:
Niacin + Statin → increased risk myopathy, hepatoxicity
Statin + Gemfibrozil → increased risk myopathy

FIGURE 1.5. Stepwise strategy for assessing and treating hypercholesterolemia in patients without known vascular disease and those with evident disease.

Management of Hypertriglyceridemia (TG > 500 mg/dl)

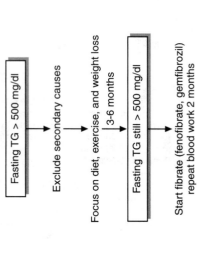

| Fasting TG > 500 mg/dl |

↓

Exclude secondary causes

↓

Focus on diet, exercise, and weight loss
3-6 months

↓

| Fasting TG still > 500 mg/dl |

↓

Start fibrate (fenofibrate, gemfibrozil)
repeat blood work 2 months

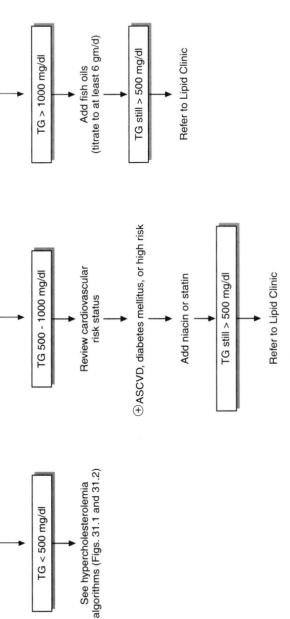

FIGURE 1.6. Strategy for the management of hypertriglyceridemia.
EVIDENCE LEVEL: C. Expert Opinion.

MANAGEMENT OF HYPERTRIGLYCERIDEMIA

13

Treatment of Hypertension

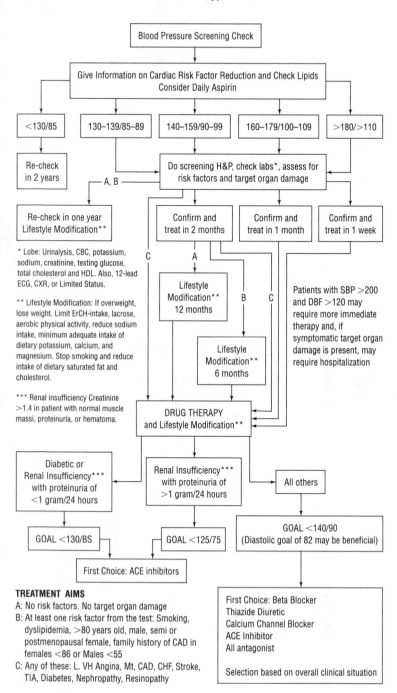

Blood Pressure Screening Check

Give Information on Cardiac Risk Factor Reduction and Check Lipids
Consider Daily Aspirin

| <130/85 | 130–139/85–89 | 140–159/90–99 | 160–179/100–109 | >180/>110 |

Re-check in 2 years

Do screening H&P, check labs*, assess for risk factors and target organ damage

A, B

Re-check in one year
Lifestyle Modification**

Confirm and treat in 2 months

Confirm and treat in 1 month

Confirm and treat in 1 week

* Lobe: Urinalysis, CBC, potassium, sodium, creatinine, testing glucose, total cholesterol and HDL. Also, 12-lead ECG, CXR, or Limited Status.

** Lifestyle Modification: If overweight, lose weight. Limit ErCH-intake, lacrose, aerobic physical activity, reduce sodium intake, minimum adequate intake of dietary potassium, calcium, and magnesium. Stop smoking and reduce intake of dietary saturated fat and cholesterol.

*** Renal insufficiency Creatinine >1.4 in patient with normal muscle massi, proteinuria, or hematoma.

C

A

Lifestyle Modification**
12 months

B

C

Lifestyle Modification**
6 months

Patients with SBP >200 and DBF >120 may require more immediate therapy and, if symptomatic target organ damage is present, may require hospitalization

DRUG THERAPY
and Lifestyle Modification**

Diabetic or Renal Insufficiency*** with proteinuria of <1 gram/24 hours

Renal Insufficiency*** with proteinuria of >1 gram/24 hours

All others

GOAL <130/BS

GOAL <125/75

GOAL <140/90
(Diastolic goal of 82 may be beneficial)

First Choice: ACE inhibitors

TREATMENT AIMS
A: No risk factors. No target organ damage
B: At least one risk factor from the test: Smoking, dyslipidemia, >80 years old, male, semi or postmenopausal female, family history of CAD in females <86 or Males <55
C: Any of these: L. VH Angina, Mt, CAD, CHF, Stroke, TIA, Diabetes, Nephropathy, Resinopathy

First Choice: Beta Blocker
Thiazide Diuretic
Calcium Channel Blocker
ACE Inhibitor
All antagonist

Selection based on overall clinical situation

Screening History and Physical for Hypertension

History/Physical	Consider
Suggestive of true paroxysms of headaches, flushing or palpitations	Pheochromocytoma workup including 24 hour urine for VMA and metanephrines (advise patient to collect urine on days with symptoms)
Suggestive of hyper/hypo-thyroidism	Check TSH
Diastolic renal bruits or abdominal bruits with unclear source, poor response to therapy, sudden onset, significant worsening in previous control, episodic pulmonary edema, renal insufficiency, or ACE intolerance	Evaluation for renal artery stenosis by MRI angiogram or aortogram. Check plasms renin and aldosterone
Delayed or absent femoral pulses, unequal brachial cuff pressures, especially in a young person	Evaluation for aortic coastation by Thoracic MRI or CT Scan
Purple striae, severe truncal obesity	Evaluate for Cushings Syndrome using 24 hour urinary free cortisol measurement or dexamethaxone suppression test
Abnormal fundoscopic exam	More intensive treatment with early follow-up to ensure at target blood pressure

Abnormal Lab Exam	Consider
Urinalysis with proteinuria or hematuria, or creatinine >1.4 mg/dl (in patient with normal muscle mass)	Evaluate for renal parenchymal disease
Fasting glucose greater than 125 mg/dl	Evaluate and treat for diabetes
Potassium <3.5 mEq/L on no diuretics	Consider primary aldosteronism. Check plasma renin and aldosterone levels. Consider satina suppression test
Calcium >10.2 mg/dl	Evaluate for hyperparathyroidism. Check PTH
CXR with cardiomegaly, Echo with LV well >1.1 cm or LV Mass Index >125 g/m^2 (male) or >110 g/m^2 (female), or 12-lead ECG with LVH by voltage criteria	More intensive treatment with early follow-up to ensure target blood pressure

---

Patients with resistant hypertension, diagnosed or potential secondary causes of hypertension, or inability to tolerate anti-hypertensive therapy may benefit from referral to a hypertension or cardiovascular specialist.

EVIDENCE LEVEL: A. References: 1. Sixth Report of the Joint National Commission on Presentation, Detection, and Treatment of High Blood Pressure, Arch Intern Med 1997; 1 57, 24 1 3-46 2. Hansson L. Zanchetti A, Camutbers SG, Dahiol B, Elmisidt D, Julius S, Menard J, Rhan KH, Wedel H, Westerling S. Effects of intensive blood-pressure lowering and low-dose aspirin in patients with hypertension; principal results of the Hypertension Optimal (HOT) randomized trief. The Lancet, 351; 1755–1762, 1998.

FIGURE 1.7. Stepwise strategy for evaluation and treatment of hypertension.

TABLE 1.8. CHARACTERISTICS OF COMMON CAUSES OF CHEST PAIN

	Duration	Quality	Provocation	Relief	Location
Effort angina	5–15 min	Visceral, pressure	Effort, emotion	Rest, NTG	Substernal, radiates
Rest angina	5–15 min	Visceral, pressure	Spontaneous	NTG	Substernal, radiates
Mitral prolapse	Minutes to hours	Visceral pressure	Spontaneous, no pattern	Time	Left anterior
Esophageal reflux	10–60 min	Visceral	Recumbency, lack of food	Food, antacid, upright position	Substernal, epigastric
Esophageal spasm	5–60 min	Visceral	Spontaneous, cold liquids, exercise	NTG	Substernal, radiates
Peptic ulcer	Hours	Visceral, burning	Lack of foods, "acid" foods	Foods, antacids	Epigastric, substernal
Biliary disease	Hours	Visceral, colic	Spontaneous, foods	Time, analgesics	Epigastric, RUQ, radiates
Cervical disease	Variable	Superficial	Head/neck movement, palpation	Time, analgesics	Chest
Musculoskeletal pain	Variable	Superficial	Movement, palpation	Time, analgesics	Multiple
Pulmonary	30+ min	Visceral, pressure	Often spontaneous	Rest, time, bronchodilator	Multiple

NTG, nitroglycerin; RUQ, right-upper quadrant.
EVIDENCE LEVEL: C. Expert Opinion.

CHARACTERISTICS OF COMMON CAUSES OF CHEST PAIN

Management of Acute Myocardial Infarction

PHARMACOLOGICAL THERAPY

MEDICATION	FIRST 24 HOURS	AFTER FIRST 24 HOURS	DISCHARGE
Aspirin	Chewed in ER (325mg)	160–325mg qd	81 mg qd indefinitely
Repert for ST ↑ or new LBBB ≤ 12 hrs of symptom onset	Front loaded 1-PA, reteplase or SK* or Primary PTCA		
Heparin	IV in t-PA, reteplase or PTCA treated pts. for large ant. MI or LV thrombus on echo: SubQ for SK or stent treated pts.	48 hours in t-PA, reteplase treated patients: SubQ heparin for all until ambulatory	Coumadin for 3–6 months if LV thrombus seen or thromboembolism, chronically for AF
Beta Blockers**	IV Meteprolol (up to 15mg in 3 divided doses) or IV Atenolol (10mg in 2 divided doses)	Oral Metoprolol 60–100mg qd or Atenolol 50–100mg qd	Oral daily indefinitely
ACE inhibitors	Start within hours of evolving MI, if no contraindications	Daily for up to 6 weeks	Longer is sx CHF or LVEF ≤ 40%
Nitroglycerin	IV for 24–28 hours if no contraindications	Only for ongoing ischemia or uncontrolled hypertension	Oral for residual ischemia
Statins			Indefinitely if TC > 160, LDL-C > 100mg/dl

NON - PHARMACOLOGICAL THERAPY

Dietary Advice		Education on low fat diet	Recommend low fat diet
Smoking	Reinforce cessation	Reinforce cessation	Referral to smoking cessation classes if desired
Exercise	Education	Hallway ambulation	Recommend regular aerobic exercise
Pre-discharge ETT	For uncomplicated pt. plan on 4–5 days	Perform pre-discharge ETT	Cath pts. with significant ischemia
Measure LVEF		ECHO or MUGA prior to d/c if no LV gram	ACE inhibitors if LVEF ≤ 40% or in-hospital CHF
Cardiac Rehabilitation		Start Exercise	Refer to rehab program near their home
Estrogen Replacement Therapy		Counsel all post menopausal women about potential benefits of ERT	Offer options of ERT

FIGURE 1.9. Systemic approach to evidence-based evaluation and treatment of acute myocardial infarction.

Patient Management

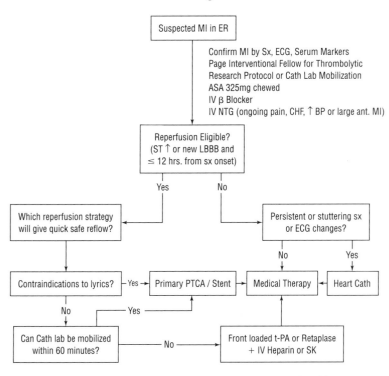

INDICATIONS FOR CARDIAC CATH:

- 1° PTCA
- Rescue for the failed thrombolysis
- Clinical conditions
  - Cardiogenic shock
  - CHF
  - Suspected mechanical complications
    eg. VSD, ruptured papillary muscle
  - Recurrent symptomatic arryhthmia
- Ischemia on pre-discharge ETT

CONTRAINDICATIONS TO THROMBOLYTICS

Absolute	Relative
Altered consciousness	Active peptic ulcer
Active internal bleeding	disease h/o
Head trauma/spinal or IC AVM/tumor	embolic or
Known prior hemorrhagic CVA	ischemic CVA
Known bleeding disorder	Pregnancy
Suspected aortic dissection	Subclavian or IJ
Persistent BP ≥ 180/110mmHg	canulation
Trauma or surgery within 2 weeks	

**Relative Contraindications to β Blockers (From card front)

Heart rate < 60 bpm	PR interval ≥ 0.24 seconds	Severe PVD
SAP < 100 mmHg	2nd or 3rd hear block	IDDM
Signs of peripheral hypoperfusion	Severe COPD	
Moderate or severe LV failure	Hx of Asthma	

*Thrombolytic Drug Dosing (From card front)

t-PA, 15 mg bolus IV, followed by 50 mg over next 30 min, followed by 35 mg over next 60 min
Retaplase, double bolus 10 IU 30 min apart
SK, 1.5 million IU infused over 60 min

EVIDENCE LEVEL: A. Reference: ACC/AHA Task Force Report on Practice Guidelines for Management of Acute MI

Biochemical Marker	Duration	Peak	Sensitivity	Specificity	Remarks
Glycogen phosphorylase BB	1 hr—unknown	unknown	Probably high	Unknown	May be released in ischemia without necrosis
Myoglobin	1–12 hrs	3–5 hrs	High (near 100%)	Low	Detected within 1 h after onset of infarction, increase with any muscle injury
Myoglobin/CAIII ratio	1–12 hrs	3–5 hrs	Probably high	Probably high	Under evaluation
Myoglobin/FABP ratio	1–12 hrs	3–5 hrs	Probably high	Possibly high	Under evaluation
CKMB/CPK ratio	12–36 hrs	20–28 hrs	High	High	Serial measurement, current WHO reference standard
TnI	8–48 + hrs	12–24 hrs	High (near 100%)	High (near 100%)	Prognostic indicator, no rise in renal failure, no cross-reaction with skeletal Tn
TnT	8–48 + hrs	12–24 hrs	High	High	Rises in renal failure, cross-reactive with skeletal Tn
LDH isoenzymes	36–72 + hrs	36–48 hrs	Low for early diagnosis	Low	Isoenzyme form improves specificity

EVIDENCE LEVEL: C. Expert Opinion.

[a] Biochemical markers for infarction/ischemia differ in temporal appearance and peak after onset of infarction and in sensitivity and specificity.

[b] Duration represented here is the approximate amount of time that a marker is present at a level of twice the upper limit of normal.

Key—duration of time that a marker is present at a level of twice the upper limit of normal; xx peak and duration of peak; CAIII, carbonic anhydrase III; FABP, fatty acid binding protein; CPK, creatine phosphokinase; TnI, troponin I; TnT, troponin T; LDH, lactate dehydrogenase.

CARDIOLOGY

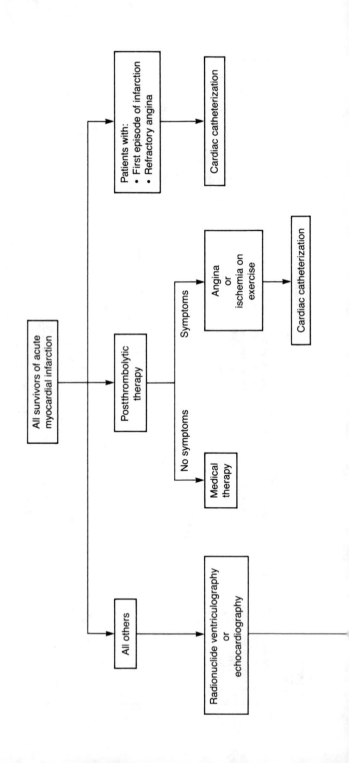

22

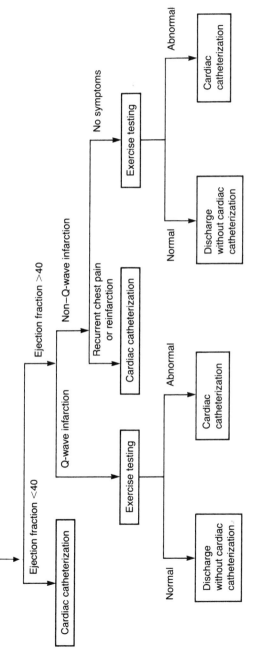

FIGURE 1.11. Protocol to be followed in determining whether patients should undergo noninvasive testing or cardiac catheterization. **EVIDENCE LEVEL: C. Expert Opinion.**

PROTOCOL FOR NONINVASIVE TESTING OR CARDIAC CATHETERIZATION

CARDIOLOGY

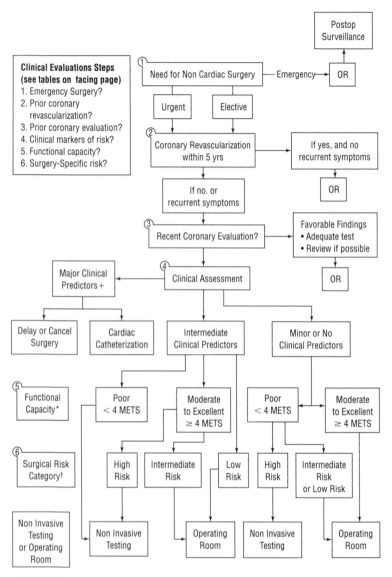

EVIDENCE LEVEL: A. Reference: Eagle KA, (Chair), Brundage BH, Chaitman BR, Ewy GA, Fleischer LA, Hertzer NR, Lappo JA, Ryan Schlant RC, Spencer WH, Spittall JA Jr, Twiss ACC/AHA Task Force Special Report Guidelines perioperative cardiovascular evaluation for noncardiac surgery. Report of the American College Cardiology/American Heart Association Task Force on Practice Guidelines. Circulation 1996:83; 1278–1317. Paul SD, Eagle KA, A Stepwise Strategy for Coronary Risk Assessment for Noncardiac Surgery. Med Clin North America, 1995:79;1241–1262

FIGURE 1.12. Stepwise approach to the pre-operative evaluation of patients being considered for non-cardiac surgery.

Table 1. Estimated Energy Requirements for Various Activities*

1 MET	4 METs
• Can you take care of yourself?	• Climb a flight of stairs or walk up a hill?
• Eat, dress or use the toilet?	• Walk on level ground at 4 mph or 6.4 km/h?
• Walk indoors around the house?	• Run a short distance?
• Walk a block or two on level ground at 2–3 mph or 3.2–4.8 km/h?	• Do heavy work around the house like scrubbing floors or lifting or moving heavy furniture?
• Do light work around the house like dusting or washing dishes?	• Participate in moderate recreational activities like golf, bowling, dancing, doubles tennis, or throwing a baseball or football?
4 METs	>10 METs
	• Participate in strenuous sports like swimming, singles tennis, football, basketball, or skiing?

Table 2. Clinical Predictors of Increased Cardiovascular Risk
(Myocardial Infarction, Congestive Heart Failure, Death)

Major
• Unstable coronary syndromes
• Recent MI with evidence of important ischemic risk by clinical symptoms or noninvasive study
• Unstable or severe angina (Canadian Class III or IV)
  Decompensated congestive heart failure
  Significant arrhythmias
• High-grade atrioventricular block
• Symptomatic ventricular arrhythmias in the presence of underlying heart disease
• Supraventricular arrhythmias with uncontrolled ventricular rate
• Severe valvular disease

Intermediate
• Mild angina pectoris (Canadian Class I or II)
• Prior myocardial infarction by history or pathological Q-waves
• Compensated or prior CHF
• Diabetes mellitus

Minor
• Advanced age
• Abnormal ECG (left ventricular hypertrophy, left bundle branch block, ST-T abnormalities)
• Rhythm other than sinus (eg. atrial fibrillation)
• Low function capacity (eg. inability to climb one flight of stairs with a bag of groceries)
• History of stroke
• Uncontrolled systemic hypertension

Table 3. Cardiac Risk Stratification for Noncardiac Surgical Procedures

Major
(Reported cardiac risk often>5%)
• Emergent major operations, particularly in the elderly
• Aortic and other major vascular
• Peripheral vascular
• Anticipated prolonged surgical procedures associated with large fluid shifts and/or blood loss

Intermediate
(Reported cardiac risk 1–5%)
• Carotid endartectomy
• Head and neck
• Intraperitoneal and intrathoracic
• Orthopedic
• Prostate

Low[†]
(Reported Cardiac Risk generally <1%)
• Endoscopic procedures
• Superficial procedure
• Cataract
• Breast

* Combined incidence of cardiac death and nonfatal myocardial infarction.
[†] Do not generally require further preoperative cardiac testing

ECG indicates electrocardiogram
* The ACC National Database Library defines recent MI as greater than 7 days but less than or equal to 1 month (30 days).
** May include stable angina in patients who are unusually sedentary.
[†] Campeau L. Grading of angina pectoris, Circulation, 1976:54

Assess Airway, Breathing, Circulation.
Perform CPR until monitor / defibrillation attached.
Confirm asystole in more than one lead.
Asystole present

↓

Continue CPR
Intubate trachea
Obtain IV access

↓

Consider and treat possible underlying causes

↓

Consider immediate transcutaneous cardiac pacing

↓

Epinephrine 1 mg IV push;
repeat every 3-5 minutes and consider escalating doses

↓

Atropine, 1 mg IV; repeat every 3-5 minutes to a total of 0.03 - 0.04 mg/kg

↓

Consider termination of resuscitation efforts

FIGURE 1.13. Algorithm for asystole and profound bradycardia. (Modified from American Heart Association. *Textbook of advanced cardiac life support,* 1997.) **EVIDENCE LEVEL: A. Reference: *Textbook of Advanced Cardiac Life Support.* American Heart Association 1997:1–24.**

Assess Airway, Breathing, Circulation
Perform CPR until monitor / defibrillation attached
Assess rhythm
PEA present

↓

Continue CPR
Intubate trachea
Obtain IV access
Assess blood flow using Doppler ultrasound, if available

↓

Consider and treat possible underlying causes

↓

Epinephrine, 1 mg IV push; repeat every 3 - 5 minutes

↓

IV volume infusion

↓

If bradycardia, give atropine 1 mg IV;
repeat every 3 - 5 minutes as needed to a total of 0.03 - 0.04 mg/kg

↓

Consider trial of pressor agent

FIGURE 1.14. Algorithm for pulseless electrical activity. (Modified from American Heart Association. *Textbook of advanced cardiac life support,* 1997.)
EVIDENCE LEVEL: A. Reference: *Textbook of Advanced Cardiac Life Support.* American Heart Association 1997:1–22.

Assess Airway, Breathing, Circulation
Perform CPR until defibrillator attached
VF/VT present

↓

Defibrillate up to 3 times if needed for persistant VF/VT
(200 joules, 200-300 J, 360 J)
Reassess rhythm

↓

Persistent or recurrent VF/VT

↓

Continue CPR
Intubate trachea
Obtain IV access

↓

Epinephrine 1 mg IV push; repeat every 3-5 min until pulse restored

↓

Defibrillate (360 J) within 30-60 sec.

↓

If persistent VF/VT, administer antiarrhythmic medication of probable benefit.
Choices: Lidocaine, amiodarone, bretylium, magnesium sulfate, procainamide, propranolol.
Sodium bicarbonate may be added if hyperkalemia,
bicarbonate-responsive drug overdose or preexisting acidosis.

↓

Defibrillate (360 J) within 30-60 sec after each dose
Pattern should be drug-shock, drug-shock if VF/VT persists.

FIGURE 1.15. Algorithm for ventricular fibrillation and pulseless ventricular tachycardia. (Modified from American Heart Association. *Textbook of advanced cardiac life support,* 1997.)
EVIDENCE LEVEL: A. Reference: *Textbook of Advanced Cardiac Life Support.* American Heart Association 1997:1–17.

Antibiotic Prophylaxis for Procedure Related Endocarditis

Structural Cardiac Conditions: Prophylaxis Recommended

High-Risk
- Prosthetic cardiac valves
- Previous endocarditis
- Cyanotic congenital heart disease
  (eg. single ventricle, transposition, tetralogy)
- Surgically corrected systemic - pulmonary
  shunts and conduits

Moderate-Risk
- Other congenital cardiac malformations (except below)
  - Acquired valvular dysfunction
    (eg. rheumatic heart disease)
  - Hypertrophic cardiomyopathy
  - Mitral valve prolapse with regurgitation
    and/or thickened leaflet

Negligible-Risk
(Prophylaxis not recommended)
- Isolated secundum ASD
- Surgical repair of ASD, VSD or PDA
  (without residue beyond 6 months)
- Previous CABG
- Mitral valve prolapse without valvular
  regurgitation
- Functional heart murmurs
- Cardiac pacemakers or defibrillators

Dental, Oral, Resp, or Esophageal procedures
- Dental: extractions, cleaning if bleeding
  anticipated periodental procedures,
  implants, root canals.
- Prophylactic cleaning of teeth or implants
  where bleeding is anticipated
- Periodontal procedures: surgery, scaling
  and root planing, probing and recall
  maintenance
- Dental implant placement and
  reimplantation of avulsed teeth
- Endontic (root canal) Instrumentation or
  surgery beyond the apex
- Respiratory
- Tonsillectomy and/or adenoidectomy
- Operations that involve respiratory
  mucosa
- Bronchoscopy with rigid broncoscope
- Esophageal
- Sclerotherapy for esophageal varices
- Esophageal stricture dialation

Prophylactic Regimens		
Situation	**Agent**	**Regimens**
Standard	Amoxicillin	2.0g orally 1 hr before
Unable to take or absorb oral meds	Ampicillin	2.0g IM or IV 30 min before
Allergic to Penicillin	Clindamycin or Caphalaxin or Cefadrxil Azithromycin or Clarithromycin	600mg PO, 1 hr before 2.0g PO, 1 hr before or 500mg PO, 1 hr before
Allergic to penicillin and unable to take oral medications	Clindamycin or Cefazolin	600mg IV within 30 min before 1.0g IM or IV within 30 min before
* Cephalosporins should not be used in individuals with immediate type hypersensitivity reaction to penicillins (urticaria, angioedema or anaphylaxis).		

EVIDENCE LEVEL: A. Reference: JAMA, June 11, 1997 - Vol 277, No 22 (p1794–1801)

FIGURE 1.16. Simplified approach to antibiotic prophylaxis for procedure related bacterial endocarditis.

CARDIOLOGY

Non Esophageal GI and GU Procedures

Prophylactic Regimens

Non Esophageal GI	Situation	Agent	Regimen
ERCP with biliary obstruction Biliary tract surgery Operations that involve intestinal mucosa	High-Risk patients	Ampicilin plus Gentamicin	Amp 2.0g IM/TV plus Gentamicin 1.5 mg/Kg (not to exceed 120mg) within 30 min of starting the procedure: 6 hrs later, Amp Ig IM/TV or Amox Ig PO.

Genitourinary Tract	Situation	Agent	Regimen
Prostatic surgery	High-Risk allergic to Amp or Amor	Vancomycin Gentamicin	Vanco 1g IV over 1–2 hrs plus Gentamicin 1.5 mg/Kg IV/IM (not to exceed 120mg) complete injection/infusion within 30 min of starting the procedure.
Cystoscopy	Moderate Risk	Amoxicillin	Amox 2.0g PO 1 hr before or Amp 2.0g IM/TV within 30 min of procedure.
Urethral dialation	Moderate-Risk allergic to Amp or Amor	Vancomycin	Vanco 1.0 g IV over 1–2 hr. complete infusion within 30 min of procedure.

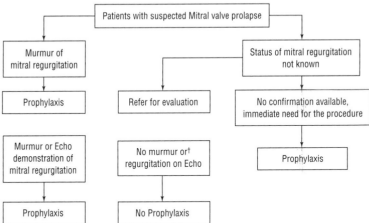

†Men > 45 yrs with MVP with intermittant murmur warrant prophylaxis

Special Circumstances

1. Patient on antibiotic normally used for endocarditis—selected drug from different class. Delay procedure 9–14 days after the completion of the antibiotic.
2. Procedures involving the infected tissues—Antibiotic directed at likely pathogen causing infection.
3. Patients on Heparin—avoid IM injections; patients on werfarin—IM is a relative contraindication.
4. Patients undergoing cardiac surgery—thorough preoperative dental evaluation; complete dental treatment before cardiac surgery.
5. Surgery for placement of prosthetic heart valves,—perioperative prophylaxis with antistaphylococcal antibiotic (usual or intravascular materials).
6. Non coronary vascular grafts—antibiotic prophylaxis for the first 6 months after procedure.

ANTIVIOTIC PROPHYLAXIS FOR PROCEDURE RELATED ENDOCARDITIS

2

GASTROENTEROLOGY

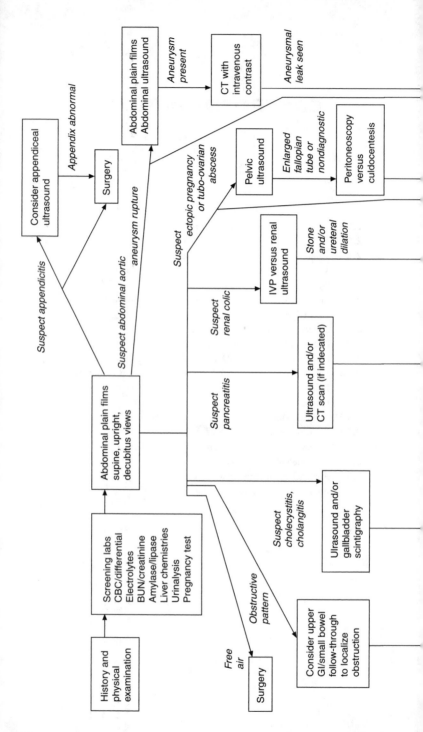

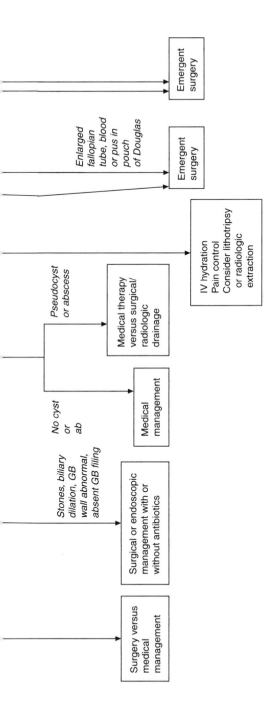

FIGURE 2.1. Evaluation of acute abdomen.
EVIDENCE LEVEL: C. Expert Opinion.

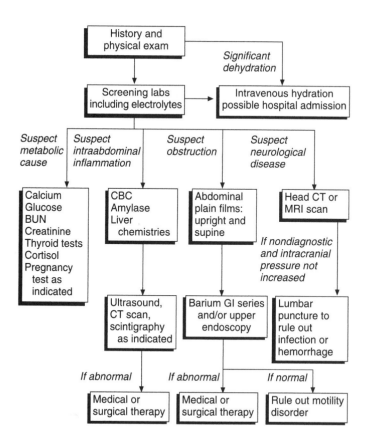

FIGURE 2.2. Evaluation of nausea and vomiting.
EVIDENCE LEVEL: C. Expert Opinion.

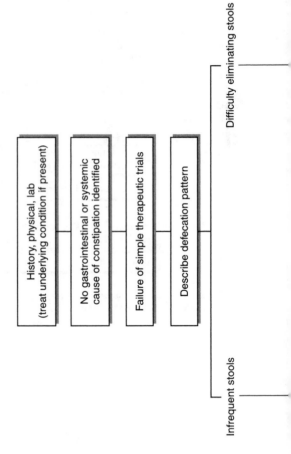

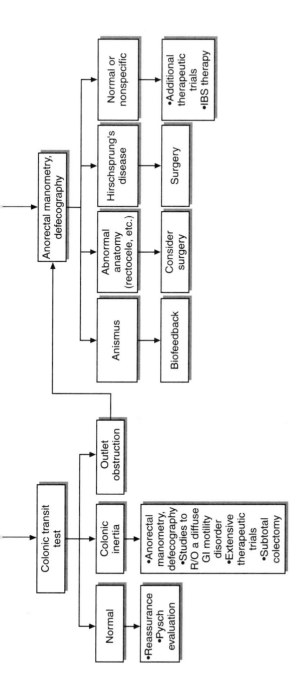

FIGURE 2.3. Algorithm for the approach to the patient with constipation.
EVIDENCE LEVEL: C. Expert Opinion.

APPROACH TO THE PATIENT WITH CONSTIPATION

39

Dysphagia

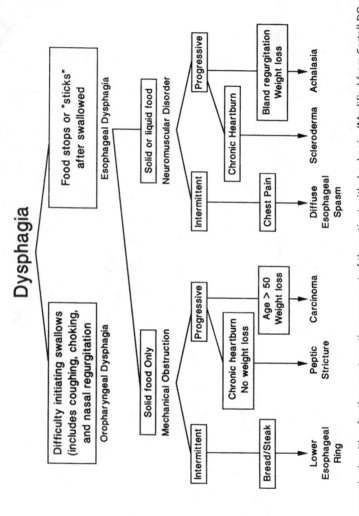

FIGURE 2.4. Diagnostic algorithm for the symptomatic assessment of the patient with dysphagia. (Modified from Castell DO, Donner MW. Evaluation of dysphagia: a careful history is crucial. *Dysphagia* 1987;2:65–71.) **EVIDENCE LEVEL: B. Reference: AGA Medical Position Statement on Management of Oropharyngeal Dysphagia. *Gastroenterology* 1999;116:452–478.**

Dysphagia

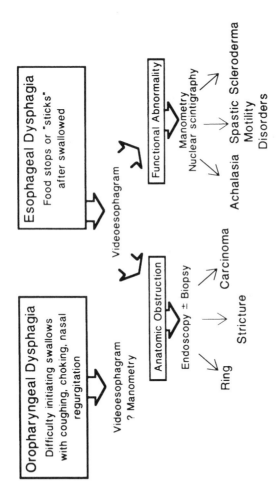

FIGURE 2.5. Algorithm for the appropriate use of diagnostic tests in evaluating the patient with dysphagia. The barium esophagogram, preferably using the video technique, is the initial diagnostic test for patients presenting with either oropharyngeal or esophageal dysphagia. **EVIDENCE LEVEL: B. Reference: AGA Medical Position Statement on Management of Oropharyngeal Dysphagia.** *Gastroenterology* **1999;116:452–478.**

SYMPTOMATIC ASSESSMENT OF PATIENT WITH DYSPHAGIA   DIAGNOSTICS IN EVALUATING PATIENT WITH DYSPHAGIA

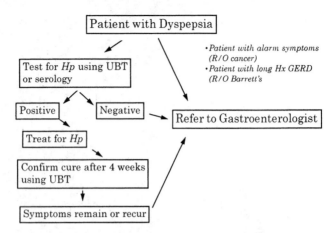

FIGURE 2.6. Clinical pathway for the treatment of patients with suspected peptic ulcer (dyspepsia) to assist in decision making regarding when to refer the patient to a gastroenterologist.
EVIDENCE LEVEL: C. Expert Opinion.

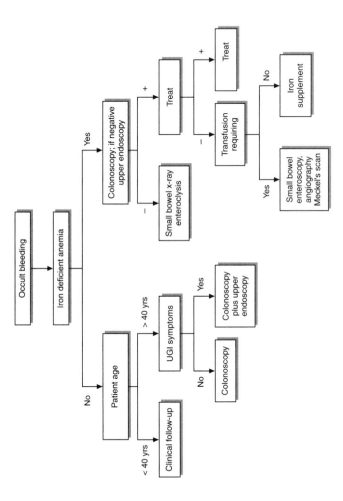

FIGURE 2.7. Evaluation of occult gastrointestinal bleeding.
EVIDENCE LEVEL: C. Expert Opinion.

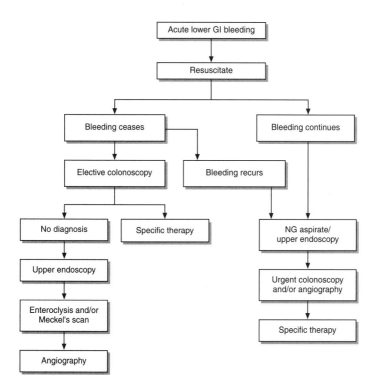

FIGURE 2.8. Evaluation of lower gastrointestinal bleeding.
EVIDENCE LEVEL: C. Expert Opinion.

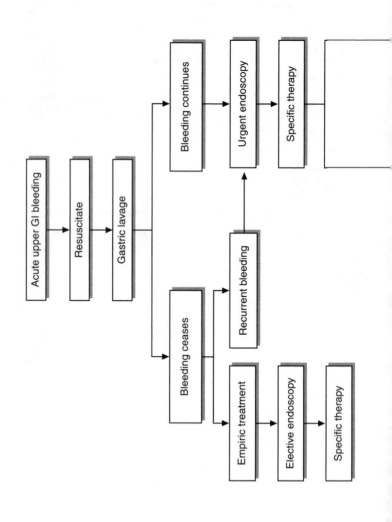

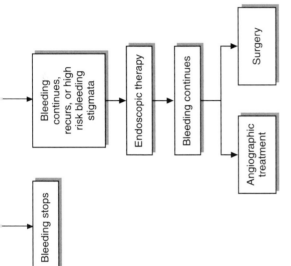

FIGURE 2.9. Evaluation of nonvariceal upper gastrointestinal bleeding.
EVIDENCE LEVEL: C. Expert Opinion.

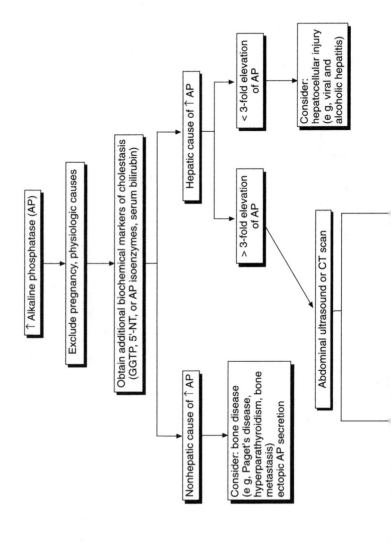

↑ Alkaline phosphatase (AP)

Exclude pregnancy, physiologic causes

Obtain additional biochemical markers of cholestasis
(GGTP, 5'-NT, or AP isoenzymes, serum bilirubin)

Nonhepatic cause of ↑ AP

Consider: bone disease
(e.g, Paget's disease,
hyperparathyroidism, bone
metastasis)
ectopic AP secretion

Hepatic cause of ↑ AP

> 3-fold elevation
of AP

< 3-fold elevation
of AP

Consider:
hepatocellular injury
(e.g, viral and
alcoholic hepatitis)

Abdominal ultrasound or CT scan

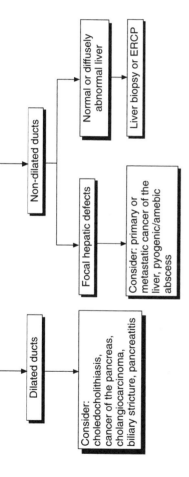

FIGURE 2.10. Diagnosing the patient with elevated serum alkaline phosphatase levels. *CT*, computed tomography; *ERCP*, endoscopic retrograde cholangiopancreatography; *GGTP*, serum γ-glutamyl transpeptidase; *5'-NT*, 5'-nucleotidase.
EVIDENCE LEVEL: C. Expert Opinion.

DIAGNOSING THE PATIENT WITH ELEVATED SERUM ALKALINE PHOSPHATASE LEVELS

TABLE 2.11. CAGE QUESTIONNAIRE[a]

Have you felt that you should **C**ut down on your drinking?
Have you felt **A**nnoyed by people criticizing your drinking?
Have you ever felt **G**uilty about your drinking?
Do you require an "**E**ye-opener" in the morning to steady yourself or get rid of a hangover?

---

[a] A score of two or more positive answers to this screening test correlates highly with alcohol abuse or dependence.

EVIDENCE LEVEL: B. Reference: Bisson J, Nadeau L, Demers A. The validity of the CAGE scale to screen for heavy drinking and drinking problems in a general population survey. *Addiction* **1999;94:715–722.**

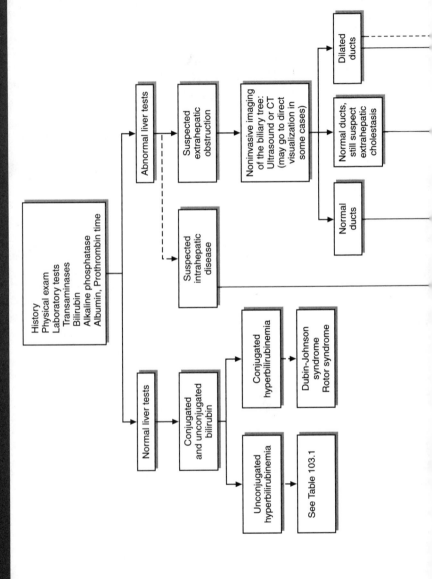

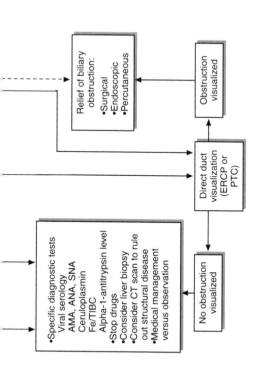

FIGURE 2.12. Evaluation for jaundice. *Dotted line,* alternative approach for certain patients. *AMA,* antimitochondrial antibody; *ANA,* antinuclear antibody; *SMA,* smooth-muscle antibody; *Fe/TIBC,* iron/total iron binding capacity.
EVIDENCE LEVEL: C. Expert Opinion.

The following content appears within the figure:

- Relief of biliary obstruction:
  - •Surgical
  - •Endoscopic
  - •Percutaneous

- Obstruction visualized

- Direct duct visualization (ERCP or PTC)

- No obstruction visualized

- Specific diagnostic tests
  - Viral serology
  - AMA, ANA, SNA
  - Ceruloplasmin
  - Fe/TIBC
  - Alpha-1-antitrypsin level
- •Stop drugs
- •Consider liver biopsy
- •Consider CT scan to rule out structural disease
- •Medical management versus observation

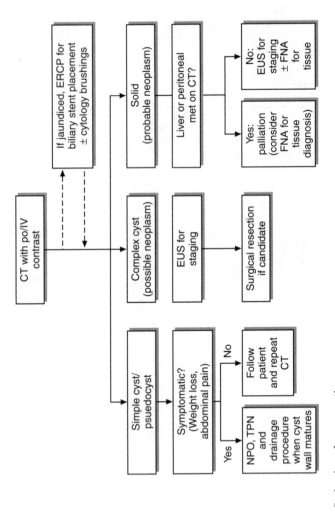

FIGURE 2.13. Evaluation of a pancreatic mass.
EVIDENCE LEVEL: C. Expert Opinion.

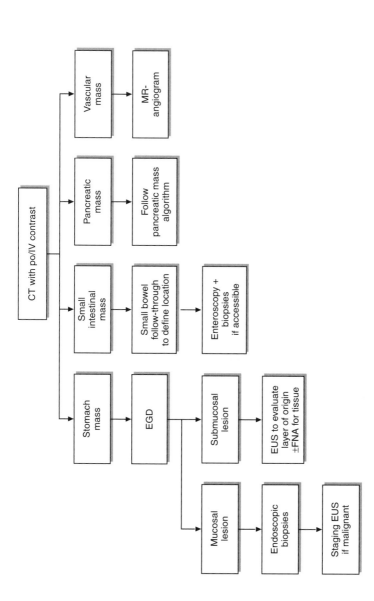

FIGURE 2.14. Evaluation of a suspected upper abdominal mass. **EVIDENCE LEVEL: C. Expert Opinion.**

EVALUATION OF A SUSPECTED UPPER ABDOMINAL MASS

EVALUATION OF A PANCREATIC MASS

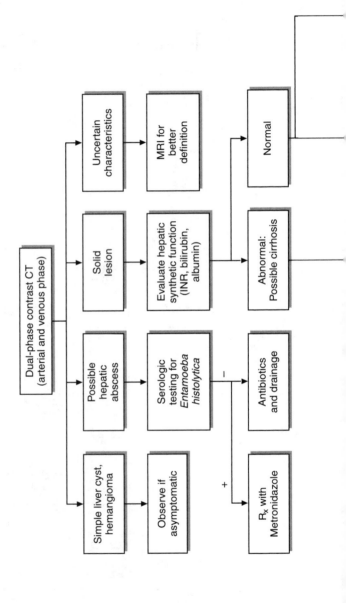

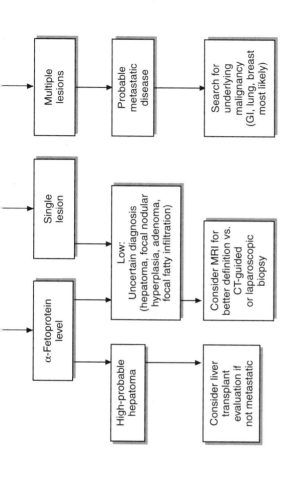

FIGURE 2.15. Evaluation of a liver mass.
EVIDENCE LEVEL: B. Reference: Saim S. Imaging of the hepatobiliary tract. *N Engl J Med* 1997;336:1889–1894.

EVALUATION OF A LIVER MASS

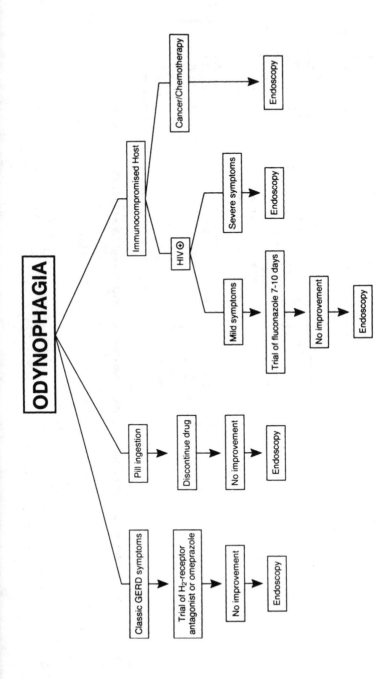

FIGURE 2.16. Approach to the patient with odynophagia. (Modified from Wilcox CM. Esophageal disease in the acquired immunodeficiency syndrome: etiology, diagnosis and management. *Am J Med* 1992;92:412–421.)
EVIDENCE LEVEL: B. Reference: Speckler SJ. AGA Technical review of treatments of patients with dysphagia. Gastroenterology

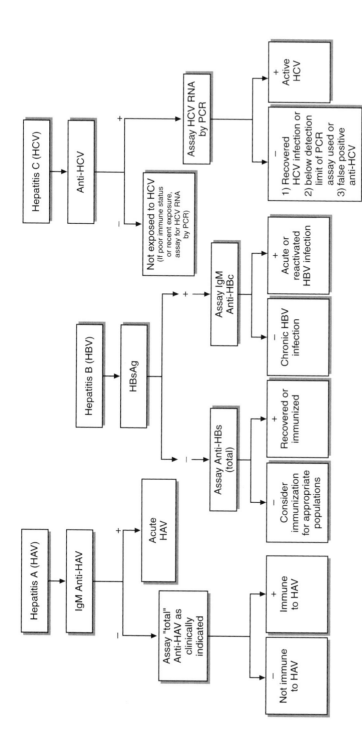

FIGURE 2.17. Approach to diagnosis of Hepatitis A infection. **EVIDENCE LEVEL: C. Expert Opinion.**

3

NEPHROLOGY

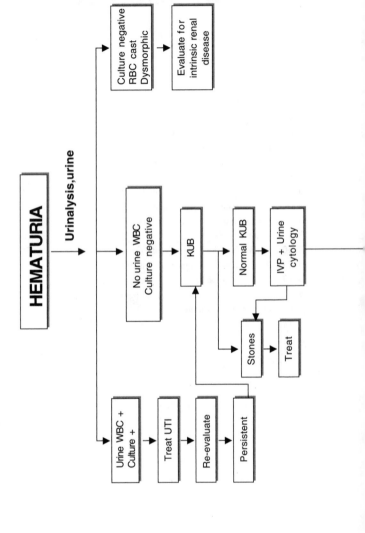

HEMATURIA

Urinalysis,urine

No urine WBC
Culture negative

Urine WBC +
Culture +

Treat UTI

Re-evaluate

Persistent

KUB

Stones

Treat

Normal KUB

IVP + Urine
cytology

Culture negative
RBC cast
Dysmorphic

Evaluate for
intrinsic renal
disease

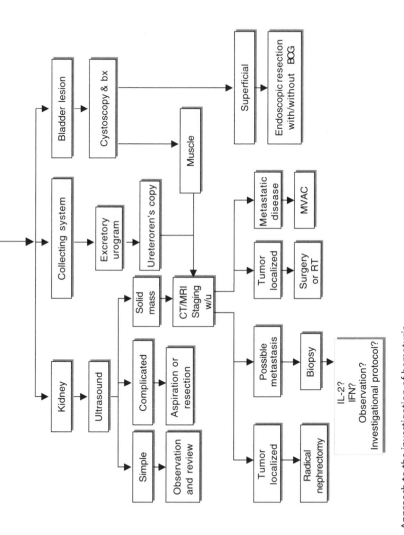

FIGURE 3.1. Approach to the investigation of hematuria.
EVIDENCE LEVEL: C. Expert Opinion.

APPROACH TO THE INVESTIGATION OF HEMATURIA

63

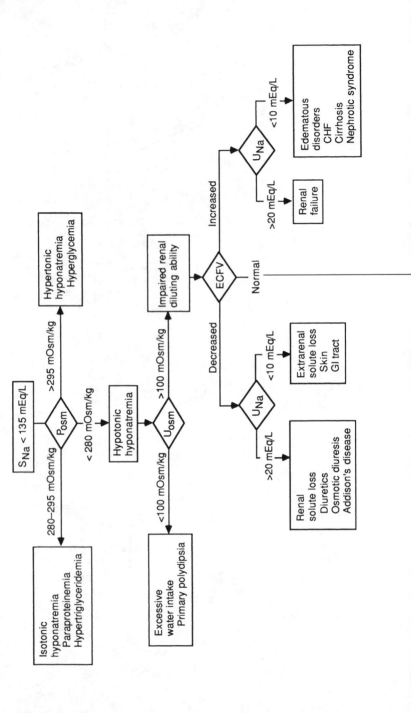

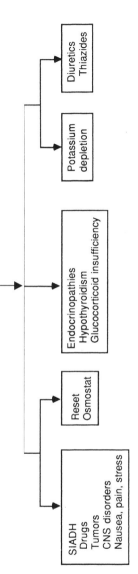

FIGURE 3.2. Approach to the patient with hyponatremia. S_{Na}, serum sodium concentration; U_{Na}, urine sodium concentration; P_{osm}, plasma osmolality; U_{osm}, urine osmolality; ECFV, extracellular fluid volume; GI, gastrointestinal; CHF, congestive heart failure; SIADH, syndrome of inappropriate antidiuretic hormone; CNS, central nervous system.
EVIDENCE LEVEL: C. Expert Opinion.

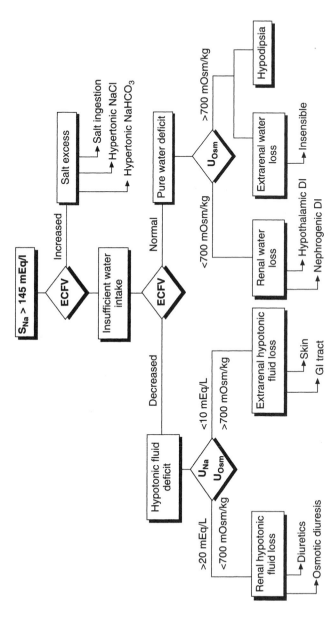

FIGURE 3.3. Approach to the patient with hypernatremia. S_{Na} and U_{Na}, serum and urine sodium concentrations, respectively; U_{Osm}, urine osmolality; ECFV, extracellular fluid volume; GI, gastrointestinal; DI, diabetes insipidus. **EVIDENCE LEVEL: C. Expert Opinion.**

APPROACH TO THE PATIENT WITH HYPERNATREMIA

67

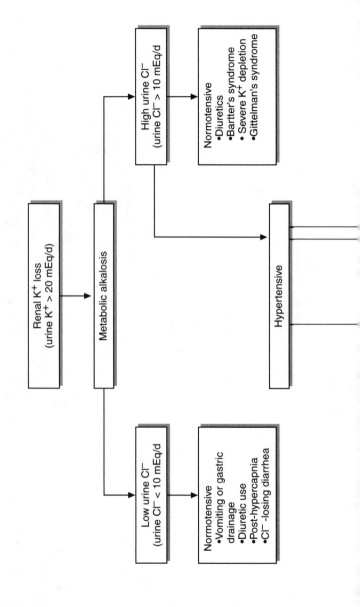

Renal K$^+$ loss
(urine K$^+$ > 20 mEq/d)

Metabolic alkalosis

High urine Cl$^-$
(urine Cl$^-$ > 10 Eq/d)

Normotensive
•Diuretics
•Bartter's syndrome
• Severe K$^+$ depletion
•Gittelman's syndrome

Low urine Cl$^-$
(urine Cl$^-$ < 10 mEq/d)

Normotensive
•Vomiting or gastric drainage
•Diuretic use
•Post-hypercapnia
•Cl$^-$ -losing diarrhea

Hypertensive

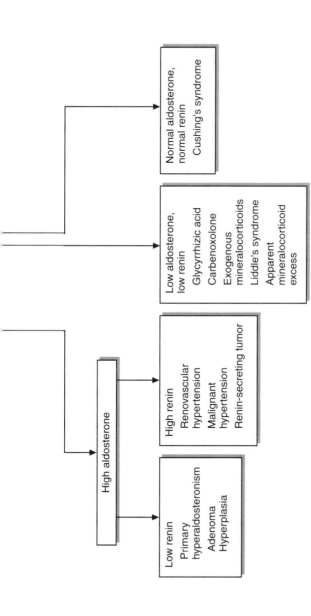

FIGURE 3.4. Differential diagnosis of hypokalemic disorders secondary to renal potassium wasting that manifest metabolic alkalosis.
EVIDENCE LEVEL: B. Reference: Seldin DW, Giebisch G, eds. *The Kidney, third edition.* Philadelphia: Lippincott Williams & Wilkins, 2000.

DIFFERENTIAL DIAGNOSIS OF HYPOKALEMIC DISORDERS

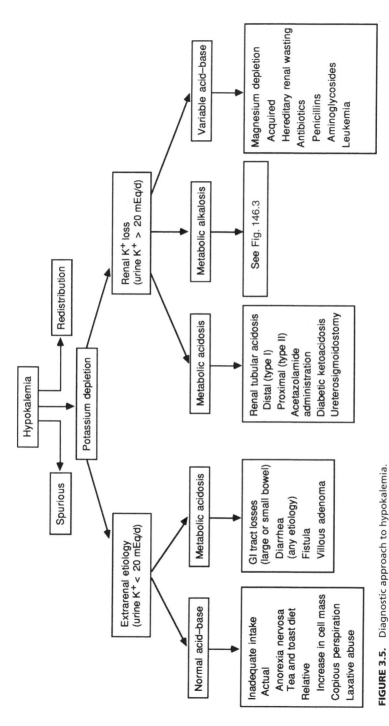

FIGURE 3.5. Diagnostic approach to hypokalemia.
EVIDENCE LEVEL: B. Reference: Seldin DW, Giebisch G, eds. *The Kidney, third edition.* **Philadelphia: Lippincott Williams & Wilkins, 2000.**

DIAGNOSTIC APPROACH TO HYPOKALEMIA

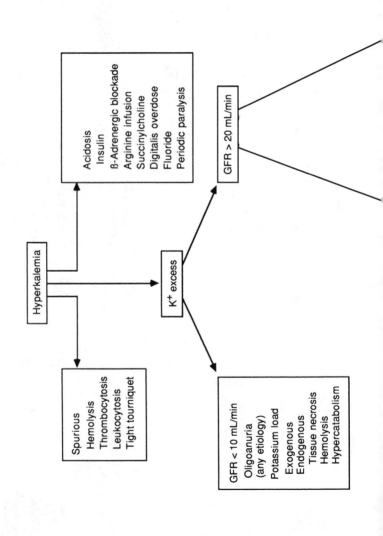

Hyperkalemia

Spurious
Hemolysis
Thrombocytosis
Leukocytosis
Tight tourniquet

Acidosis
Insulin
β-Adrenergic blockade
Arginine infusion
Succinylcholine
Digitalis overdose
Fluoride
Periodic paralysis

K⁺ excess

GFR > 20 mL/min

GFR < 10 mL/min
Oligoanuria
(any etiology)
Potassium load
    Exogenous
    Endogenous
        Tissue necrosis
        Hemolysis
        Hypercatabolism

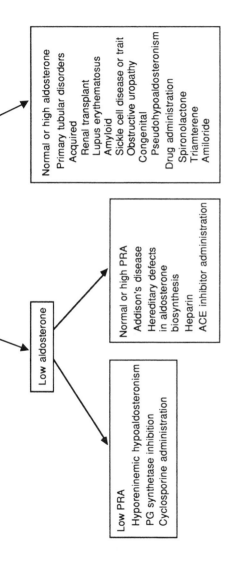

Low aldosterone

Low PRA
Hyporeninemic hypoaldosteronism
PG synthetase inhibition
Cyclosporine administration

Normal or high PRA
Addison's disease
Hereditary defects
in aldosterone
biosynthesis
Heparin
ACE inhibitor administration

Normal or high aldosterone
Primary tubular disorders
Acquired
Renal transplant
Lupus erythematosus
Amyloid
Sickle cell disease or trait
Obstructive uropathy
Congenital
Pseudohypoaldosteronism
Drug administration
Spironolactone
Triamterene
Amiloride

FIGURE 3.6. Diagnostic approach to hyperkalemia. GFR, glomerular filtration rate; PRA, plasma renin activity; PG, prostaglandin; ACE, angiotensin-converting enzyme.
EVIDENCE LEVEL: B. Reference: Weiner ID, Wingo CS. Hyperkalemia: a potential silent killer. *J Am Soc Nephrol* 1998;9:1535–1543.

DIAGNOSTIC APPROACH TO HYPERKALEMIA

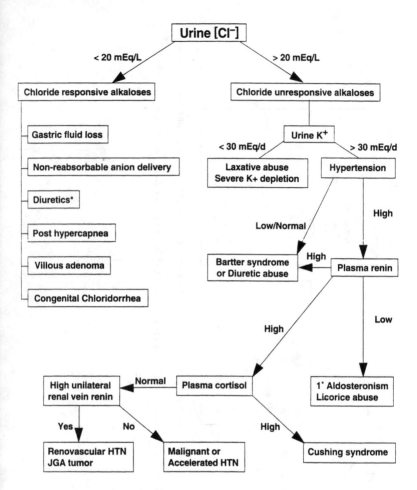

FIGURE 3.7. Diagnostic approach to metabolic alkalosis based on urine chloride and potassium concentrations.
EVIDENCE LEVEL: C. Expert Opinion.

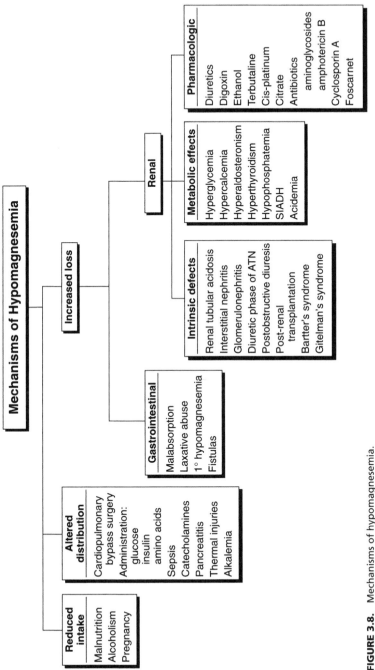

FIGURE 3.8. Mechanisms of hypomagnesemia.
EVIDENCE LEVEL: C. Expert Opinion.

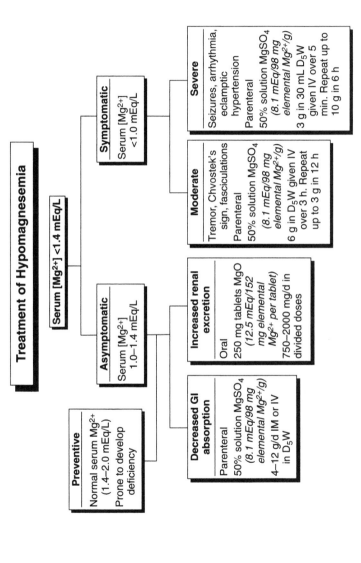

FIGURE 3.9. Treatment of hypomagnesemia.
EVIDENCE LEVEL: C. Expert Opinion.

TREATMENT OF HYPOMAGNESEMIA

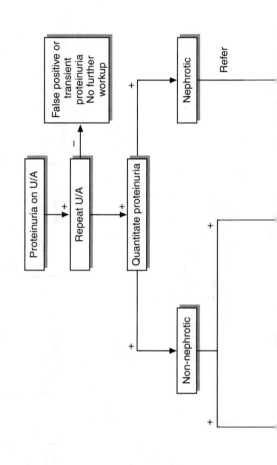

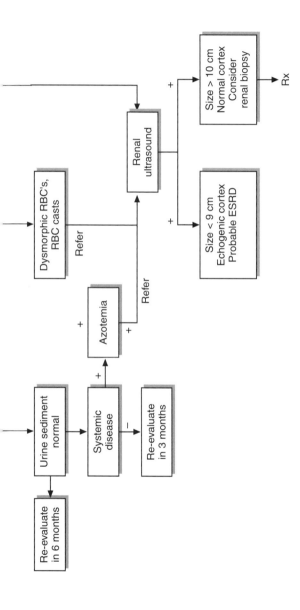

FIGURE 3.10. Approach to the evaluation of proteinuria in the adult. Urinalysis (U/A). Refer indicates where referral to a nephrologist is appropriate. Rx indicates points at which therapy can be initiated, as indicated in the text.
EVIDENCE LEVEL: B. Reference: Giatras I, Lau J, Levey AS. Effect of angiotensin-converting-enzyme inhibitors on the progression of nondiabetic renal disease: a meta-analysis of randomized trials. Angiotensin-Converting-Enzyme Inhibitor and Progressive Renal Disease Study Group. *Ann Int Med* 1997;127:337-345.

APPROACH TO THE EVALUATION OF PROTEINURIA IN THE ADULT

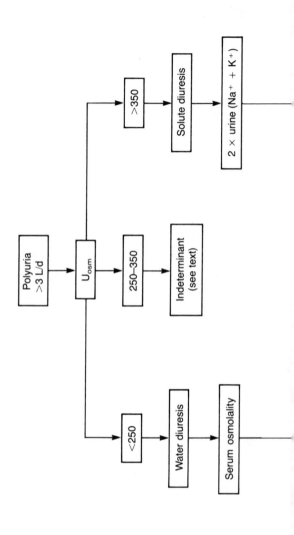

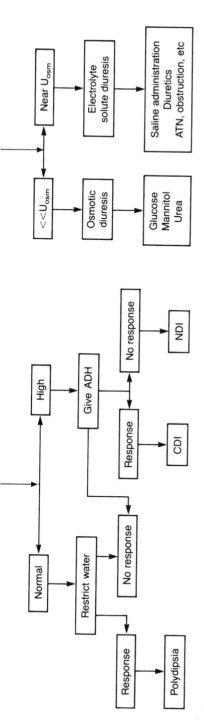

FIGURE 3.11. Approach to the diagnosis of polyuria. U_{osm}, urine osmolality; ADH, antidiuretic hormone; ATN, acute tubular necrosis; CDI, central diabetes insipidus; NDI, nephrogenic diabetes insipidus.
EVIDENCE LEVEL: C. Expert Opinion.

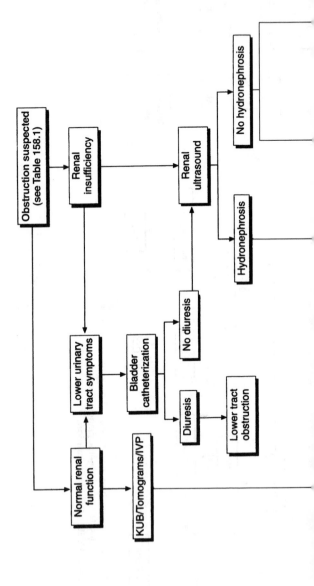

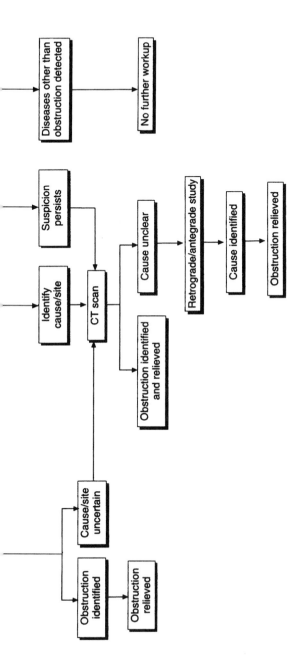

FIGURE 3.12. Approach to the patient with suspected urinary obstruction.
EVIDENCE LEVEL: C. Expert Opinion.

APPROACH TO THE PATIENT WITH SUSPECTED URINARY OBSTRUCTION

83

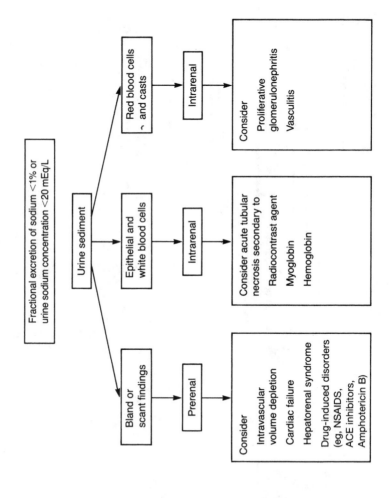

Fractional excretion of sodium <1% or urine sodium concentration <20 mEq/L

Urine sediment

Bland or scant findings

Prerenal

Consider

Intravascular volume depletion

Cardiac failure

Hepatorenal syndrome

Drug-induced disorders (eg, NSAIDS, ACE inhibitors, Amphotericin B)

Epithelial and white blood cells

Intrarenal

Consider acute tubular necrosis secondary to

Radiocontrast agent

Myoglobin

Hemoglobin

Red blood cells and casts

Intrarenal

Consider

Proliferative glomerulonephritis

Vasculitis

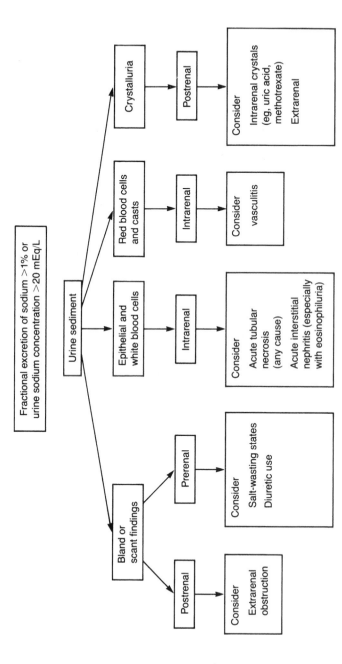

FIGURE 3.13. Use of urinary indexes and findings in the approach to the diagnosis of acute renal failure. NSAIDs, nonsteroidal anti-inflammatory drugs; ACE, angiotensin-converting enzyme.
EVIDENCE LEVEL: C. Expert Opinion.

USE OF URINARY INDEXES AND FINDINGS IN THE APPROACH TO THE DIAGNOSIS OF ACUTE RENAL FAILURE

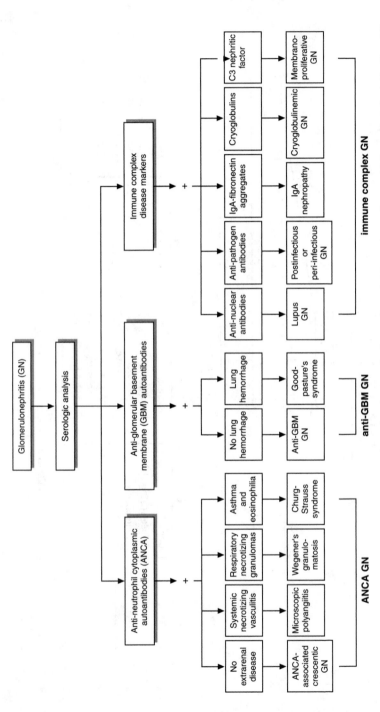

FIGURE 3.14. Diagram depicting the serologic analysis of patients with glomerulonephritis. *ANCA*, anti-neutrophil cytoplasmic antibodies; *GN*, glomerulonephritis; *GBM*, glomerular basement membrane. (Modified from Jennette JC, Falk RJ. Diagnosis and management of glomerulonephritis

4

RHEUMATOLOGY, ALLERGY, AND DERMATOLOGY

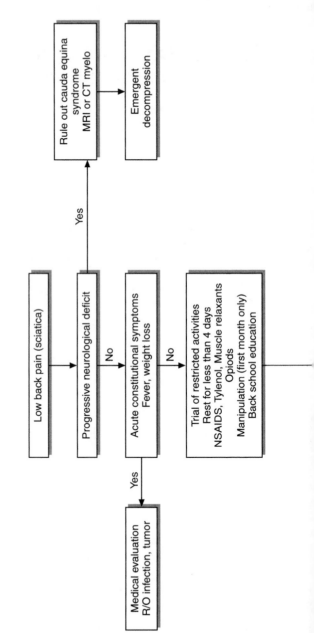

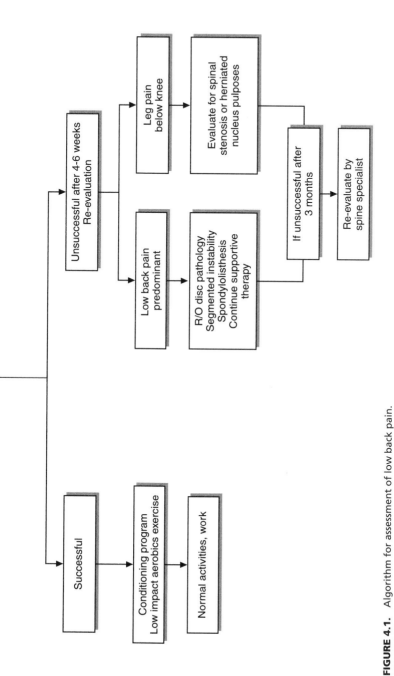

FIGURE 4.1. Algorithm for assessment of low back pain.
EVIDENCE LEVEL: B. Reference: Mooney V. Treating low back pain with exercise. *J Musculoskeletal Med* **1995;12:24–36.**

ASSESSMENT OF LOW BACK PAIN

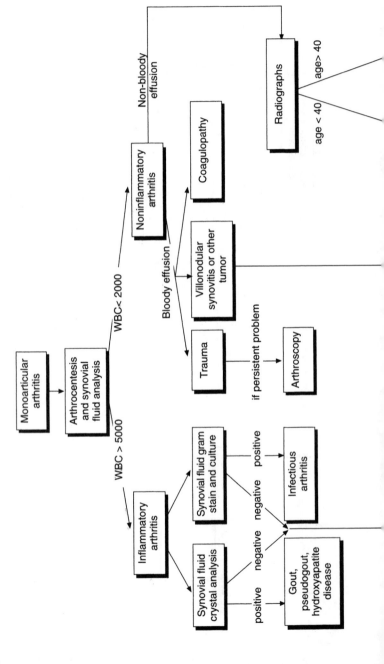

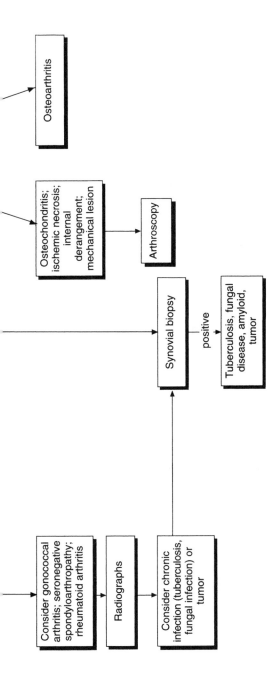

FIGURE 4.2. The flowchart shows the steps in determining whether monarticular arthritis is inflammatory or noninflammatory. **EVIDENCE LEVEL: A. Reference: Guidelines for the initial evaluation of the adult patient with acute musculoskeletal symptoms. American College of Rheumatology Ad Hoc Committee on Clinical Guidelines.** *Arthritis Rheum* **1996;39:1–8.**

MONARTICULAR ARTHRITIS

Source of data	Rheumatoid arthritis	Systemic lupus erythematosus	Ankylosing spondylitis	Gout
History and physical exam	Symmetrical polyarthritis Morning stiffness	Multisystem disease	Back pain Axial involvement	Recurrent attacks
Blood tests	Latex test + in approx. 80% Elevated ESR in 50 – 60%	ANA-screening + in >99% DNA antibodies + in 60 – 75%	Approx. 90% of patients are HLA-B27	Uric acid elevated in 75 – 90%
Radiographs	Demineralization Erosions Joint space narrowing	Generally non-destructive	Sacroiliitis Vertebral squaring	Erosions Cysts
Synovial fluid	Inflammation, WBC > 10,000	Mild inflammation	Inflammation WBC 5 – 20,000	Negatively birefringent crystals

Source of data	Osteoarthritis	Fibromyalgia	Scleroderma	Polymyositis
History and physical exam	Pain ± swelling ± limited motion	Chronic pain "all over" No swollen joints Muscle spasm	Skin tightness dorsum of hand Facial skin tightening	Muscle weakness ± pain
Blood tests	Nonspecific abnormalities	No abnormalities may have +ANA (2-5%); uric acid >8.0(2-5%)	+ANA, up to 90% with Hep-2 cells	CPK elevated in 80% +ANA in 33%
Radiographs	Joint space narrowing Osteophytes	No severe abnormalities (may have cervical osteoarthritis)	± Pulomary fibrosis ± Esophageal dysmotility ± Calcinosis	Not helpful
Synovial fluid	Non-inflammatory WBC < 10,000	None	Not specific	Not specific

FIGURE 4.3. Diagnosis of rheumatic diseases. Clinical data from different sources, with the source of the most valuable data boxed. *ANA*, antinuclear antibodies; *WBC*, white blood cell count.
EVIDENCE LEVEL: C. Expert Opinion.

DIAGNOSIS OF RHEUMATIC DISEASES

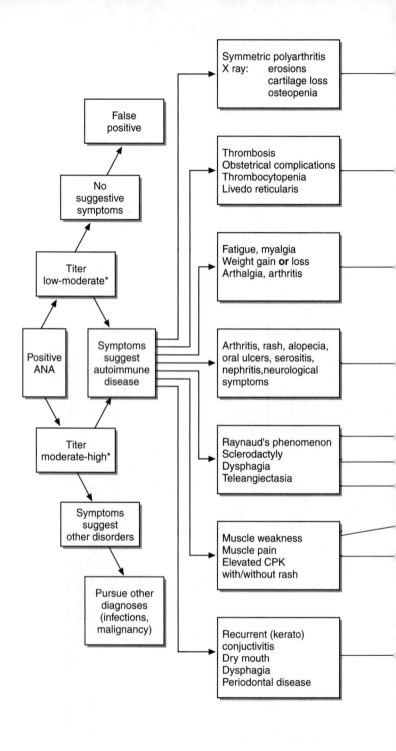

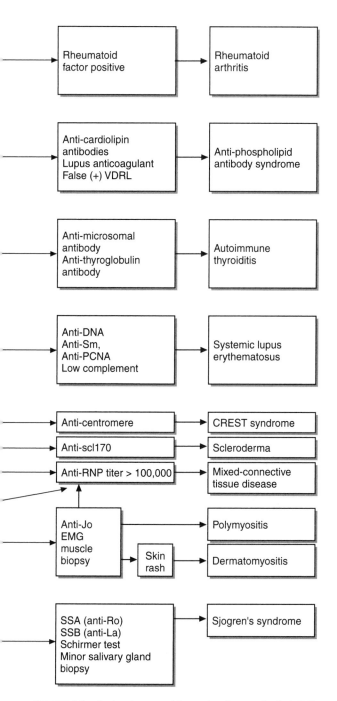

FIGURE 4.4. Evaluating a positive antinuclear antibody (ANA) result.
EVIDENCE LEVEL: C. Expert Opinion.

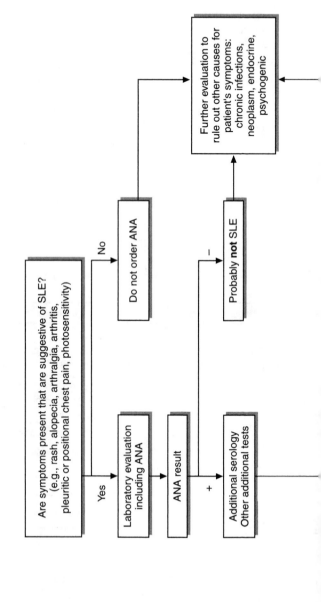

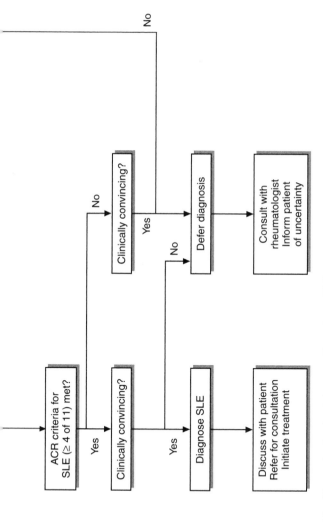

FIGURE 4.5. Diagnosis of systemic lupus erythematosus (SLE).
EVIDENCE LEVEL: C. Expert Opinion.

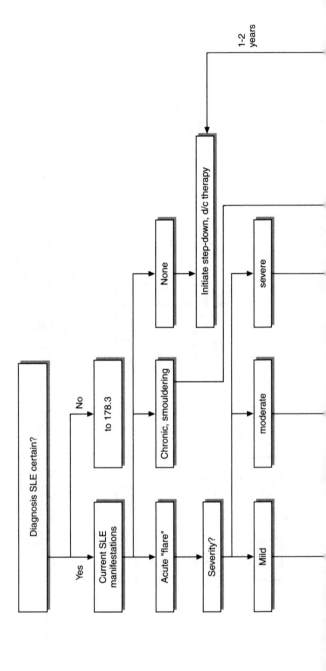

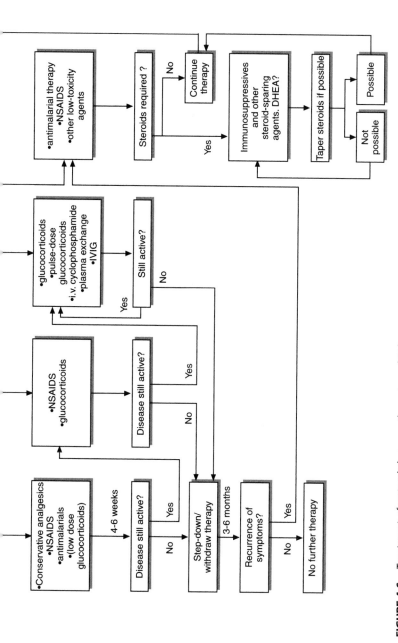

FIGURE 4.6. Treatment of systemic lupus erythematosus (SLE). **EVIDENCE LEVEL: C. Expert Opinion.**

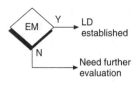

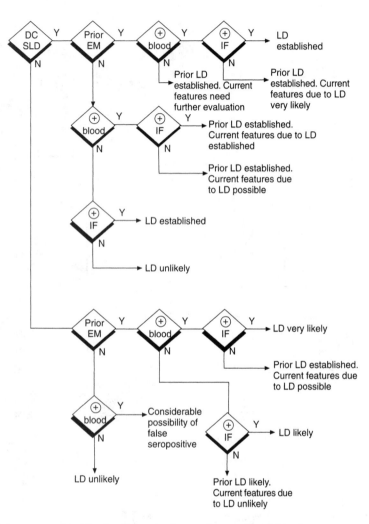

FIGURE 4.7. Algorithm for diagnosis of Lyme disease. +blood, blood test containing antibodies to *Borrelia burgdorferi;* DCSLD, defined clinical syndrome of Lyme disease (Table 183.2); EM, erythema migrans; +IF, inflammatory fluid (synovial or spinal fluid) containing antibodies to *Borrelia burgdorferi.*
EVIDENCE LEVEL: A. Reference: Nadelman RB, Wormser GP. Erythema migrans and early Lyme disease. *Am J Med* **1995;98:15S–24S.**

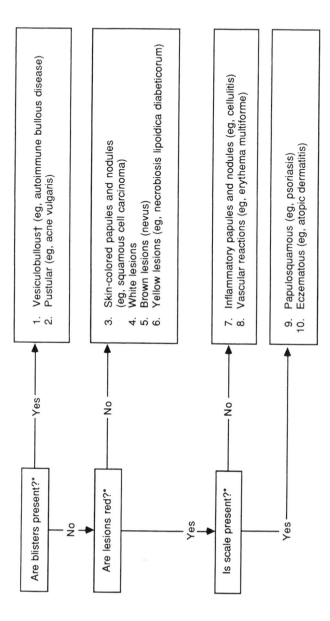

FIGURE 4.8. Problem-oriented dermatologic algorithm. Only one example is taken from each category. Please refer to the text for an expanded list of diagnoses. (Adapted from Lynch PJ. *Dermatology for the house officer*. Baltimore: Williams & Wilkins, 1982.)
EVIDENCE LEVEL: C. Expert Opinion.

Are blisters present?*

No ↓

Are lesions red?*

No →

1. Vesiculobullous† (eg, autoimmune bullous disease)
2. Pustular (eg, acne vulgaris)

Yes →

3. Skin-colored papules and nodules (eg, squamous cell carcinoma)
4. White lesions
5. Brown lesions (nevus)
6. Yellow lesions (eg, necrobiosis lipoidica diabeticorum)

Is scale present?*

Yes ↓

No →

7. Inflammatory papules and nodules (eg, cellulitis)
8. Vascular reactions (eg, erythema multiforme)

9. Papulosquamous (eg, psoriasis)
10. Eczematous (eg, atopic dermatitis)

Initial Assessment
History, physical examination
Cardiovascular, respiratory, cutaneous manifestations

Initial Treatment
Trendelenburg position
Aqueous epinephrine (1:1000) 0.3-0.5 mL SC every 5-30 min
Diphenhydramine 25-50 mg PO, IM, IV every 6 hr
Supplemental O_2 4-6 L nasal cannula
Volume expansion (IV isotonic saline, lactated Ringers)

Resolution
Discharge with followup
(see text)

Reassessment

Persistent Symptoms

Corticosteroids-methylprednisolone 1-2 mg/kg IV every 6 hr

Persistent Hypotension
Supplemental O_2
Monitor cardiac rhythm, pulse, blood pressure
Repeat aqueous epinephrine
Continue volume expansion (1 L every 15-30 min)
and consider human serum albumin, plasma or
other colloid solutions

Persistent Airway Obstruction

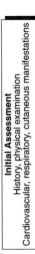

TREATMENT OF ANAPHYLAXIS

Laryngeal Edema
Supplemental O$_2$
Monitor cardiac rhythm, pulse, blood pressure, pulse oximetry
Repeat aqueous epinephrine
Consider nebulized racemic epinephrine 0.5 mL (2.25% soln) in 2.5 mL NS
Emergency tracheostomy, cricothyrotomy

Bronchospasm
Supplemental O$_2$
Monitor cardiac rhythm, pulse, blood pressure, pulse oximetry, ABG
Repeat aqueous epinephrine
Nebulized β-agonist
Metaproterenol 0.3 mL (5% soln) in 2.5 mL NS
Albuterol 0.5 mL (0.5% soln) in 2.5 mL NS

Aminophylline infusion 6 mg/kg loading dose in 100cc D$_5$W over 20 min continuous infusion 0.9 mg/kg/hr (monitor serum levels)
Repeat corticosteroids
Intubation, assisted ventillation as necessary

Epinephrine infusion 1.0 mL 1:1000 aqueous epinephrine in 250 mL D$_5$W (4 μg/mL) at 1-4 μg/min
Pregnant patient: consider ephedrine 25-50 mg IV
Patient on β-blocker: isoproterenol 1 mg in 500 mL D$_5$W (2 μg/mL) at 0.1 μg/kg/min. May double every 15 min

Dopamine infusion 200 mg in 500 mL D$_5$W (400 μg/mL) at 5-20 μg/kg/min

Norepinephrine infusion 4 mg in 1000 mL D$_5$W (4 μg/mL) at 0.5-1.0 μg/kg/min

Glucagon 1 mg IV may be useful in refractory cases. A continuous infusion 1 mg in 1000 mL D$_5$W at 5-15 mL/min may be necessary for several hours
Cimetidine 300 mg IV or ranitidine 50 mg IV over 5 min may be used in refractory cases. Caution: avoid cimetidine in patients receiving β-blocking agents or theophylline preparations
Continue IV fluids & corticosteroids

FIGURE 4.9. Treatment of anaphylaxis.
EVIDENCE LEVEL: B. References: Atkinson TP. Anaphylaxis. *Clin Allergy* 1992;76:8. Bechner BS. Anaphylaxis. *N Engl J Med* 1991;324:1785.

5

ONCOLOGY AND HEMATOLOGY

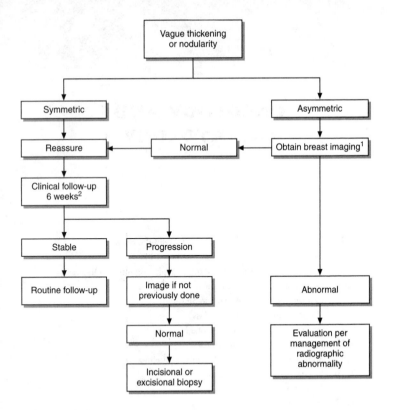

1. Age < 30: Consider ultrasound
   Age ≥ 30: Obtain diagnostic mammogram ± ultrasound
2. Or one week post menses in premenopausal women

FIGURE 5.1. Algorithm for the assessment of thickening or nodularity of the breast. The objective is to focus the invasive diagnostic assessment on asymmetric findings and to provide adequate short-term follow-up care to ensure stability of symmetric findings.
EVIDENCE LEVEL: C. Expert Opinion.

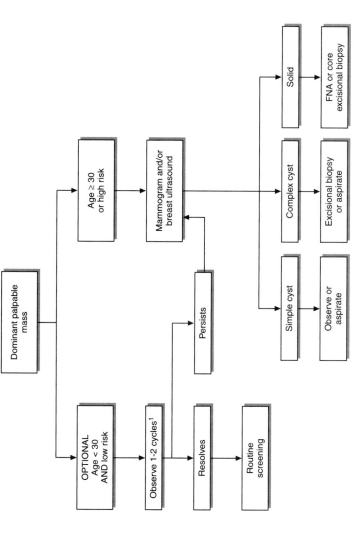

1. Re-examine day 5-7 of menstrual cycle

FIGURE 5.2. Algorithm for assessment of a palpable dominant breast mass. The objective of this evaluation is to differentiate benign and malignant causes with the triad of physical examination, imaging, and tissue sampling. **EVIDENCE LEVEL: C. Expert Opinion.**

THICKENING OR NODULARITY OF BREAST

PALPABLE DOMINANT BREAST MASS

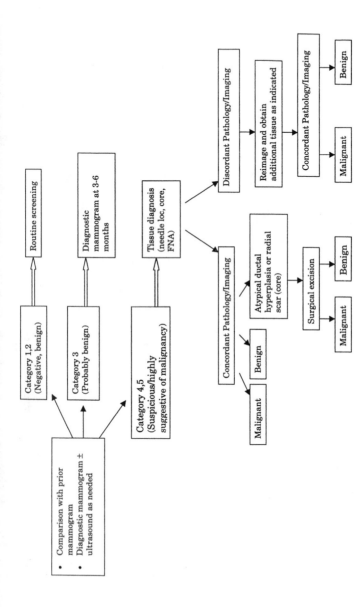

FIGURE 5.3. Algorithm for assessment after abnormal mammographic results are obtained. The objective of this evaluation is to help identify lesions that have moderate or high probability of being malignant and to assist in the procurement of accurate tissue diagnosis. (Adapted from *National Comprehensive Cancer Network breast cancer screening guidelines*, version 1. Rockledge, PA: National Comprehensive Cancer Network, 1999, with permission.)

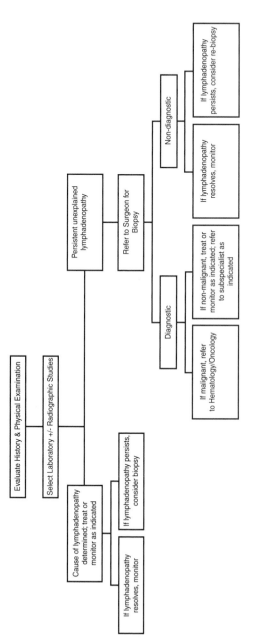

FIGURE 5.4. Algorithm for the evaluation of lymphadenopathy. Empiric antibiotics or corticosteroids should not be given. If biopsy performed, co-ordinate with the surgeon and pathologist to ensure proper processing of specimen.
EVIDENCE LEVEL: C. Expert Opinion.

Flowchart content:

- Evaluate History & Physical Examination
- Select Laboratory +/- Radiographic Studies
  - Cause of lymphadenopathy determined; treat or monitor as indicated
    - If lymphadenopathy resolves, monitor
    - If lymphadenopathy persists, consider biopsy
  - Persistent unexplained lymphadenopathy
    - Refer to Surgeon for Biopsy
      - Diagnostic
        - If malignant, refer to Hematology/Oncology
        - If non-malignant, treat or monitor as indicated; refer to subspecialist as indicated
      - Non-diagnostic
        - If lymphadenopathy resolves, monitor
        - If lymphadenopathy persists, consider re-biopsy

ASSESSMENT AFTER ABNORMAL MAMMOGRAPHIC RESULTS/EVALUATION OF LYMPHADENOPATHY

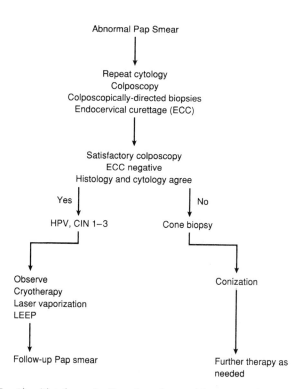

FIGURE 5.5. Algorithm for evaluation of an abnormal Pap smear. *LEEP,* Loop electrosurgical excision procedure. (Modified from Giuntoli RL, Atkinson BF, Ernst CS, et al. *Atkinson's correlative atlas of colposcopy, cytology, and histopathology.* Philadelphia: JB Lippincott, 1987:233.)
EVIDENCE LEVEL: B. Reference: Cervical cytology: evaluation and management of abnormalities. *ACOG Technical Bulletin* 1993;183:1–8.

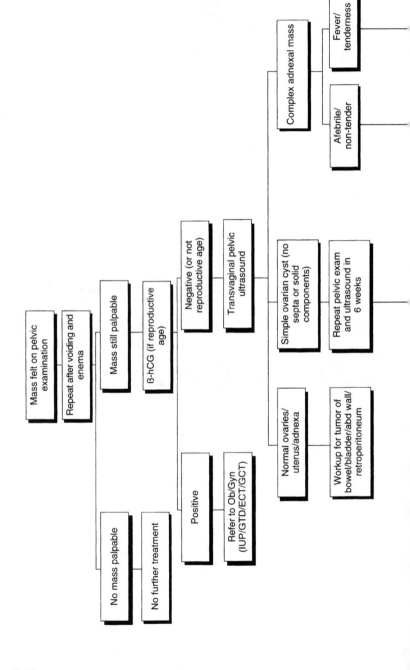

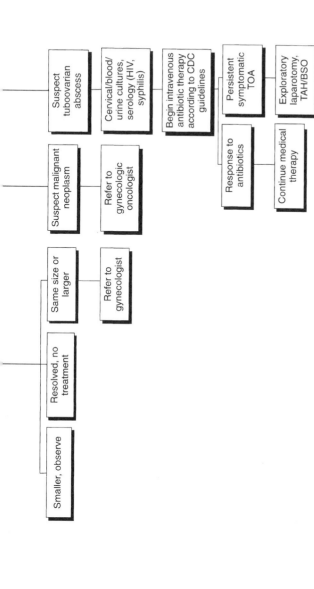

FIGURE 5.6. Algorithm for management of an adnexal mass. *β-hCG,* β-human chorionic gonadotropin; *CDC,* Centers for Disease Control and Prevention; *ECT,* ectopic pregnancy; *GCT,* germ cell tumor; *GTD,* gestational trophoblastic disease; *HIV,* human immunodeficiency virus; *IUP,* intrauterine pregnancy; *TAH,* total abdominal hysterectomy; *TOA,* tuboovarian abscess. **EVIDENCE LEVEL: C. Expert Opinion.**

MANAGEMENT OF AN ADNEXAL MASS

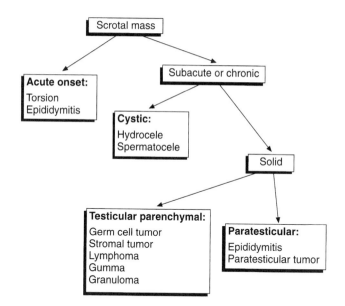

FIGURE 5.7. Differential diagnosis of a scrotal mass.
EVIDENCE LEVEL: C. Expert Opinion.

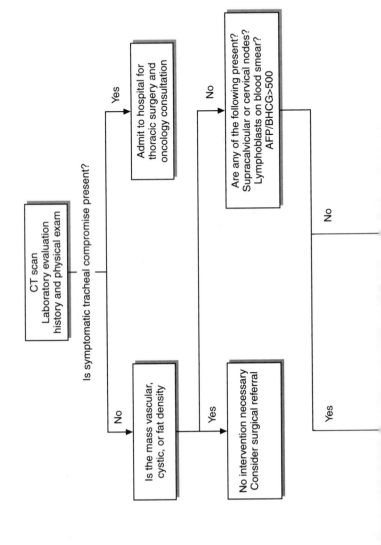

CT scan
Laboratory evaluation
history and physical exam

Is symptomatic tracheal compromise present?

Yes

Admit to hospital for thoracic surgery and oncology consultation

No

Are any of the following present?
Supraclavicular or cervical nodes?
Lymphoblasts on blood smear?
AFP/BHCG>500

No

Is the mass vascular, cystic, or fat density

Yes

No intervention necessary
Consider surgical referral

No

Yes

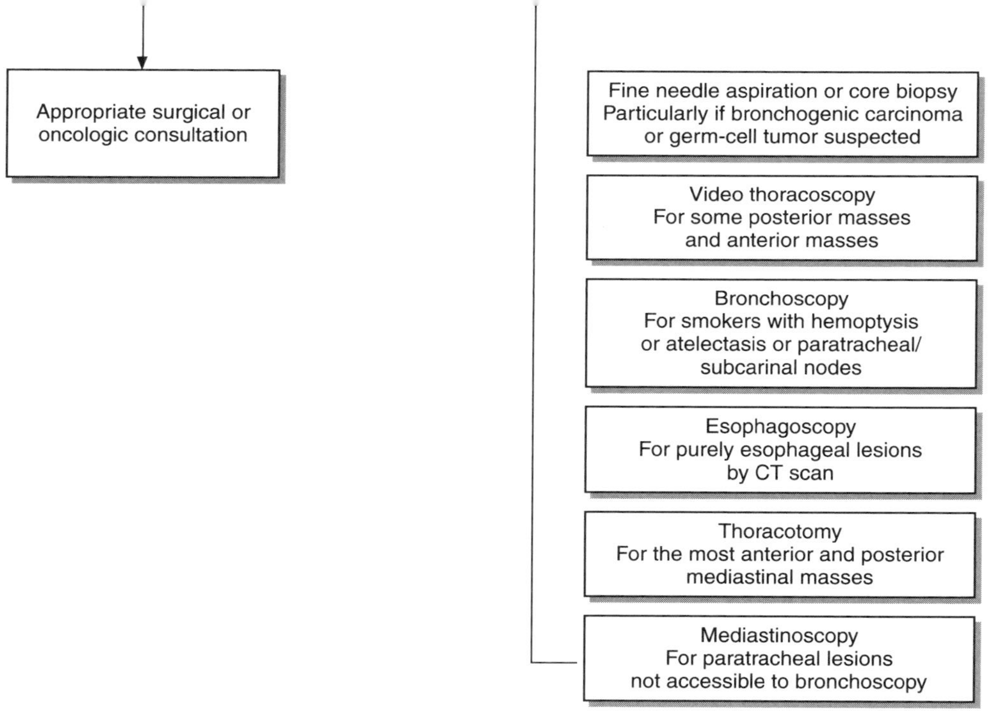

Appropriate surgical or
oncologic consultation

Fine needle aspiration or core biopsy
Particularly if bronchogenic carcinoma
or germ-cell tumor suspected

Video thoracoscopy
For some posterior masses
and anterior masses

Bronchoscopy
For smokers with hemoptysis
or atelectasis or paratracheal/
subcarinal nodes

Esophagoscopy
For purely esophageal lesions
by CT scan

Thoracotomy
For the most anterior and posterior
mediastinal masses

Mediastinoscopy
For paratracheal lesions
not accessible to bronchoscopy

FIGURE 5.8. Algorithm for evaluation of mediastinal masses. *AFP,* α-fetoprotein; *BHCG,* β-human chorionic gonadotropin; *CT,* computed tomography.
EVIDENCE LEVEL: C. Expert Opinion.

EVALUATION OF MEDIASTINAL MASSES

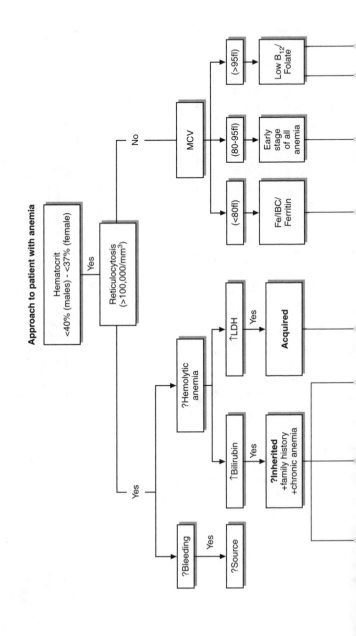

Approach to patient with anemia

Hematocrit
<40% (males) - <37% (female)

Reticulocytosis
(>100,000/mm³)

Yes

No

MCV

(<80fl)
Fe/IBC/
Ferritin

(80-95fl)
Early
stage
of all
anemia

(>95fl)
Low B₁₂/
Folate

Yes

?Bleeding
Yes
?Source

?Hemolytic
anemia

↑Bilirubin
Yes
?Inherited
+family history
+chronic anemia

↑LDH
Yes
Acquired

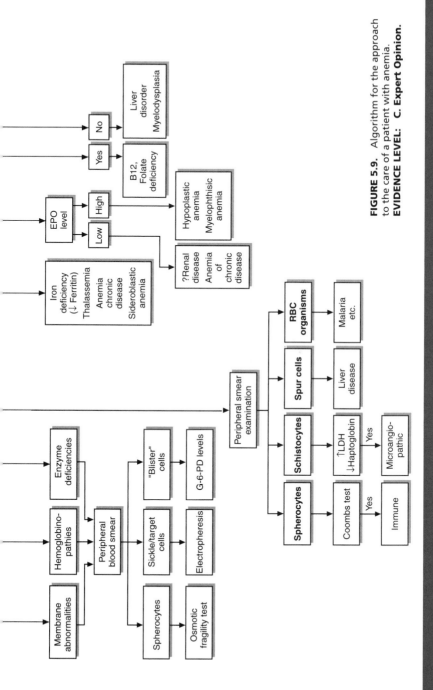

FIGURE 5.9. Algorithm for the approach to the care of a patient with anemia. **EVIDENCE LEVEL: C. Expert Opinion.**

APPROACH TO THE CARE OF A PATIENT WITH ANEMIA

119

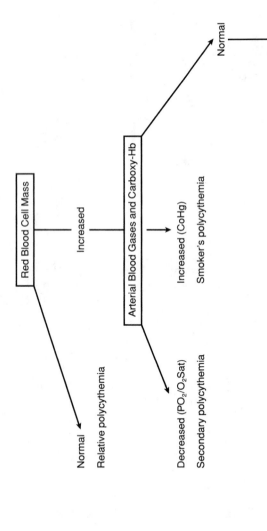

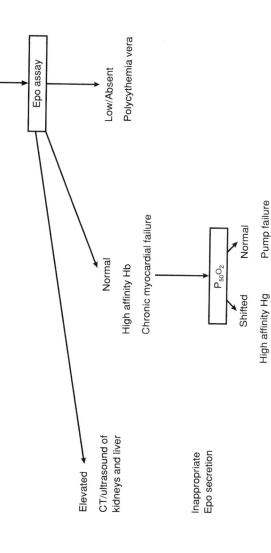

FIGURE 5.10. Algorithm for evaluation of patient with an elevated hemoglobin level. Carboxyhemoglobin is measured only for smokers or when there is potential industrial exposure. Bone marrow culture to separate normal EPO-dependent growth from EPO-independent growth in polycythemia vera is of value, but relatively unavailable. A patient with a normal EPO level and no other findings should be considered for $P_{50}O_2$ measurement to identify very rare high-affinity hemoglobin, more than 40 of which are recognized. Long-standing myocardial failure also can produce these findings.
EVIDENCE LEVEL: C. Expert Opinion.

EVALUATION OF PATIENT WITH AN ELEVATED HEMOGLOBIN LEVEL

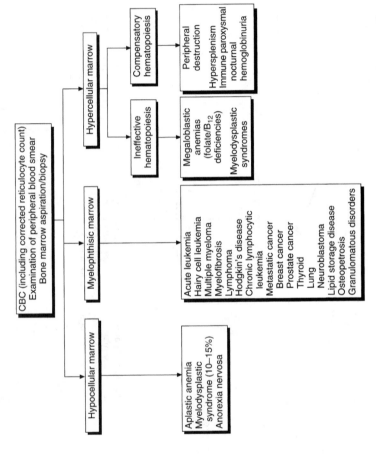

FIGURE 5.11. Algorithm for the evaluation of pancytopenia.
EVIDENCE LEVEL: C. Expert Opinion.

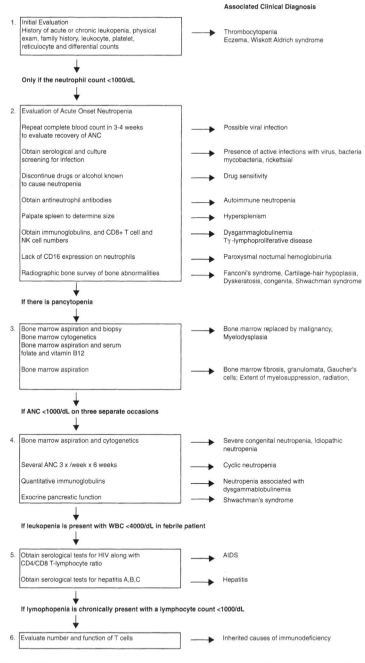

Associated Clinical Diagnosis

1. Initial Evaluation
History of acute or chronic leukopenia, physical
exam, family history, leukocyte, platelet,
reticulocyte and differential counts

→ Thrombocytopenia
Eczema, Wiskott Aldrich syndrome

Only if the neutrophil count <1000/dL

2. Evaluation of Acute Onset Neutropenia

Repeat complete blood count in 3-4 weeks
to evaluate recovery of ANC

→ Possible viral infection

Obtain serological and culture
screening for infection

→ Presence of active infections with virus, bacteria
mycobacteria, rickettsial

Discontinue drugs or alcohol known
to cause neutropenia

→ Drug sensitivity

Obtain antineutrophil antibodies

→ Autoimmune neutropenia

Palpate spleen to determine size

→ Hypersplenism

Obtain immunoglobulins, and CD8+ T cell and
NK cell numbers

→ Dysgammaglobulinemia
Tγ-lymphoproliferative disease

Lack of CD16 expression on neutrophils

→ Paroxysmal nocturnal hemoglobinuria

Radiographic bone survey of bone abnormalities

→ Fanconi's syndrome, Cartilage-hair hypoplasia,
Dyskeratosis, congenita, Shwachman syndrome

If there is pancytopenia

3. Bone marrow aspiration and biopsy
Bone marrow cytogenetics
Bone marrow aspiration and serum
folate and vitamin B12

→ Bone marrow replaced by malignancy,
Myelodysplasia

Bone marrow aspiration

→ Bone marrow fibrosis, granulomata, Gaucher's
cells; Extent of myelosuppression, radiation,

If ANC <1000/dL on three separate occasions

4. Bone marrow aspiration and cytogenetics

→ Severe congenital neutropenia, Idiopathic
neutropenia

Several ANC 3 x /week x 6 weeks

→ Cyclic neutropenia

Quantitative immunoglobulins

→ Neutropenia associated with
dysgammablobulinemia

Exocrine pancreatic function

→ Shwachman's syndrome

If leukopenia is present with WBC <4000/dL in febrile patient

5. Obtain serological tests for HIV along with
CD4/CD8 T-lymphocyte ratio

→ AIDS

Obtain serological tests for hepatitis A,B,C

→ Hepatitis

If lymophopenia is chronically present with a lymphocyte count <1000/dL

6. Evaluate number and function of T cells

→ Inherited causes of immunodeficiency

FIGURE 5.12. Algorithm for the evaluation of a patient with leukopenia. *ANC,*
absolute neutrophil count; *WBC,* white blood cell count.
**EVIDENCE LEVEL: B. Reference: Dr. Laurence A. Boxer. Guidelines for
evaluation for patients with neutropenia: Severe Chronic Neutropenia International Registry Guidelines.**

123

6

INFECTIOUS DISEASES

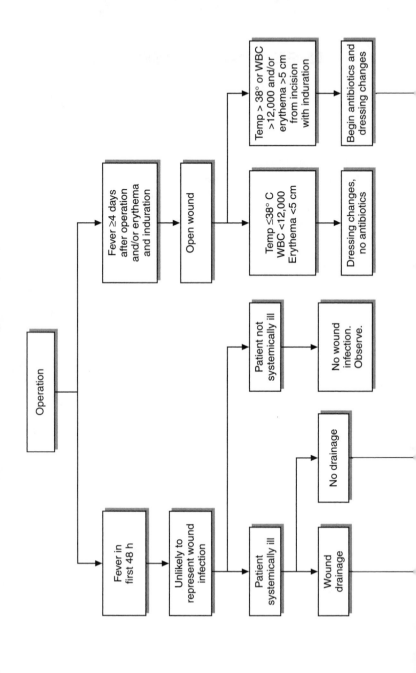

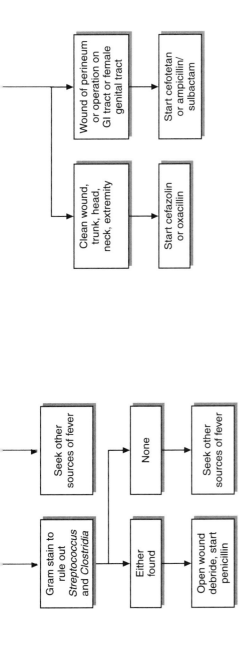

FIGURE 6.1. Diagnosis and treatment of postoperative infection. **EVIDENCE LEVEL: C. Expert Opinion.**

TABLE 6.2.   ANTIMICROBIAL THERAPY FOR INFECTIVE ENDOCARDITIS[a]

Microorganism	Suggested Regimen[b]	Comments
Penicillin-susceptible streptococci (viridans streptococci and S. bovis with MIC ≤0.1 µg/mL)	Aqueous crystalline penicillin G, 12–18 million U/24 hr for 4 weeks or Ceftriaxone, 2 g i.m./i.v. q day for 4 weeks or Aqueous crystalline penicillin G, 12–18 million U/24 hr, plus gentamicin, 1 mg/kg i.m./i.v. q 8 hr—both for 2 weeks[c]	Avoid aminoglycosides in patients older than 65 years and in those with impaired renal or eighth cranial nerve function. Substitute vancomycin, 30 mg/kg i.v. per 24 hr in two equally divided doses for 4 weeks, for penicillin in patients with immediate hypersensitivity to penicillin.[d]
Streptococci relatively resistant to penicillin G (MIC >0.1 µg/mL and <0.5 µg/mL)	Aqueous crystalline penicillin G, 18 million U/24 hr for 4 weeks, plus gentamicin, 1 mg/kg i.m./i.v. q 8 hr, for first 2 weeks[c]	Substitute cefazolin (or other first-generation cephalosporin) for penicillin in patients with non-life-threatening penicillin allergy. Substitute vancomycin, 30 mg/kg i.v. per 24 hr in two equally divided doses, for penicillin in patients with immediate hypersensitivity to penicillin[d]
Enterococci, nutritionally variant streptococci, and streptococci with penicillin MIC >0.5 µg/mL[e]	Aqueous crystalline penicillin G, 18–30 million U/24 hr (or ampicillin, 12 g/24 hr), plus gentamicin, 1 mg/kg i.m./i.v. q 8 hr—both for 4–6 weeks[c]	Substitute vancomycin, 30 mg/kg i.v. per 24 hr, in two equally divided doses for penicillin or ampicillin in patients with immediate hypersensitivity to penicillin. Cephalosporins are not acceptable alternatives.[d]
Penicillin-susceptible staphylococci (confirm with negative assay for β-lactamase production)	Aqueous crystalline penicillin G, 12–18 million U/24 hr for 4–6 weeks	Substitute cefazolin (or other first generation cephalosporin) for penicillin in patients with non-life-threatening penicillin allergy. Substitute vancomycin, 30 mg/kg i.v. per 24 hr, in two equally divided doses in patients with immediate hypersensitivity to penicillin.[d]

β-lactamase-producing, oxacillin-susceptible staphylococci	Nafcillin or oxacillin, 2 g i.v. q 4 hr for 4–6 weeks, with optional gentamicin, 1 mg/kg i.m./i.v. q 8 hr for first 3–5 days[c,f]	Substitute cefazolin (or other first-generation cephalosporin) for penicillin in patients with non-life-threatening penicillin allergy. Substitute vancomycin, 30 mg/kg i.v. per 24 hr in two equally divided doses, for nafcillin of oxacillin in patients with immediate hypersensitivity to penicillin.[d]
Oxacillin-resistant staphylococci	Vancomycin, 30 mg/kg i.v. q 24 hr in two equally divided doses for 4–6 weeks[d]	
HACEK group	Ceftriaxone, 2 g i.m./i.v. q day for 4 weeks or Ampicillin, 12 g/24 hr, plus gentamicin, 1 mg/kg i.m./i.v. q 8 hr—both for 4 weeks[c]	Do not use ampicillin if isolate produces β-lactamase
Culture-negative	Aqueous crystalline penicillin G, 18–30 million U/24 hr (or ampicillin, 12 g/24 hr) for 6 weeks, plus gentamicin, 1 mg/kg i.m./i.v. q 8 hr for 2 weeks	

MIC, minimal inhibitory concentration; HACEK group, *Haemophilus* species, *Actinobacillus actinomycetemcomitans, Cardiobacterium hominis, Eikenella corrodens,* and *Kingella* species.

[a] Suggested dosages are for patients with normal renal function. Table applies to native valve endocarditis. For patients with streptococcal endocarditis in the context of a prosthetic valve or other prosthetic material, use the regimen for enterococci and treat for 6 weeks. For staphylococcal prosthetic valve endocarditis, treat for at least 6 weeks with nafcillin, oxacillin, or vancomycin (depending on susceptibility) plus rifampin, 300 mg orally 1 8 hr, and include gentamicin as dosed above for the first 2 weeks.

[b] Aqueous crystalline penicillin G and ampicillin can be given either by continuous infusion or in six equally divided doses over 24 hr.

[c] Gentamicin dose is based on ideal body weight and should not exceed 80 mg. During therapy, further adjustments should be based on serum drug levels. Peak level of approximately 3 µg/mL is desirable.

[d] Vancomycin dose is based on ideal body weight. Vancomycin dosage should not exceed 2 g/24 hr unless serum drug levels are monitored. Peak serum level of 30–45 µg/mL is desirable.

[e] All enterococci causing endocarditis must be tested for antimicrobial susceptibility. Regimens suggested for enterococci in this table assume the isolate does not possess high-level resistance to penicillin, vancomycin, or gentamicin.

[f] Intravenous drug users who have uncomplicated tricuspid infective endocarditis due to oxacillin-susceptible *S. aureus* and no evidence of left-sided disease can be treated with nafcillin or oxacillin, 2 g i.v. q 4 hr, plus gentamicin, 1 mg/kg i.m./i.v. q 8 hr, both for 2 weeks. Vancomycin is not recommended as an alternative to nafcillin or oxacillin in 2-week regimens.

EVIDENCE LEVEL: A. Reference: Wilson WR, Karchmer AW, Dajani AS, et al. Antibiotic treatment of adults with infective endocarditis due to streptococci, enterococci, staphylococci, and HACEK microorganisms. *JAMA* 1995;274:1706–1713.

ANTIMICROBIAL THERAPY FOR INFECTIVE ENDOCARDITIS

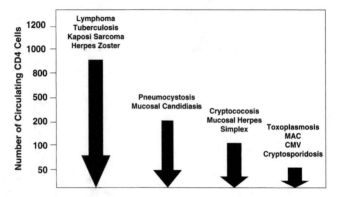

FIGURE 6.3. Typical relationship of clinical manifestations to CD4 count in HIV-infected patients.

EVIDENCE LEVEL: C. Expert Opinion.

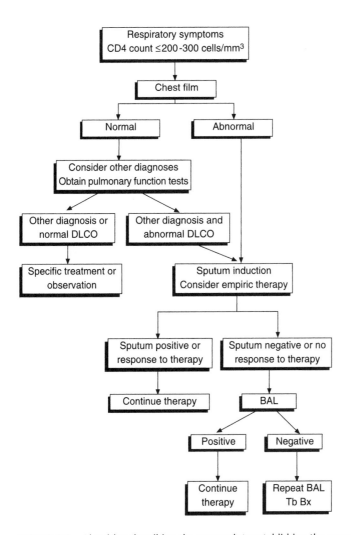

FIGURE 6.4. Algorithm describing the approach to establishing the cause of respiratory symptoms in patients with HIV infection. DLCO, diffusing capacity for carbon monoxide; BAL, bronchoalveolar lavage; Tb Bx, transbronchial lung biopsy. **EVIDENCE LEVEL: B. Hopewell PC, Masur H.** *Pneumocystis carinii* pneumonia: current concepts. In: Sande MA, Volberding PA, eds. *The medical management of AIDS,* fourth ed. Philadelphia: WB Saunders, 1995:367, with permission.

| TABLE 6.5 | PRINCIPLES OF THERAPY OF HIV INFECTION (NIH PANEL) |

Principle 1:

HIV replication leads to immune system damage and development of AIDS. HIV infection is always harmful. Long-term survival free of immune system dysfunction is rare.

Principle 2:

Plasma HIV RNA levels reflect the magnitude of HIV replication and its associated rate of CD4+-lymphocyte count decline. CD4+-lymphocyte counts indicate the current level of immune system damage. Periodic measurement of plasma HIV RNA level and CD4+-lymphocyte count is needed to assess risk for disease progression and to determine the need to initiate or alter antiretroviral therapy.

Principle 3:

Rates of disease progression vary among HIV-infected persons. Treatment decisions should be individualized based on risk of progression as indicated by plasma HIV RNA levels and CD4+-lymphocyte counts.

Principle 4:

Maximum achievable suppression of HIV replication should be the goal of therapy. The use of combinations of antiretroviral agents to suppress HIV replication to below the level of detection of plasma HIV RNA assays decreases the potential for selection of drug-resistant HIV variants.

Principle 5:

Durable suppression of HIV replication is most likely with the simultaneous initiation of combinations of antiretroviral agents with which the patient has not been previously treated and that are not cross-resistant with agents previously used.

Principle 6:

Each of the antiretroviral agents used in combination should be used according to the optimum dosages and frequencies.

Principle 7:

Any change in antiretroviral therapy decreases future therapeutic options due to the limited number of agents and significant cross-resistance between specific agents.

Principle 8:

Women should receive optimum antiretroviral therapy regardless of pregnancy.

Principle 9:

These same principles apply to children, adolescents, and adults.

Principle 10:

Acute primary HIV infection should be treated with combination antiretroviral therapy to suppress viral replication to below the level of detection of plasma HIV RNA assays.

Principle 11:

All HIV-infected persons should be considered infectious, even if the plasma HIV RNA level is below the level of detection. Counseling against activities associated with HIV transmission should continue.

EVIDENCE LEVEL: A. Reference: Report of the NIH panel to define the principles of therapy for HIV infection. *MMWR Recommendations and Reports* 1998;47:1–41.

7

PULMONARY AND CRITICAL CARE MEDICINE

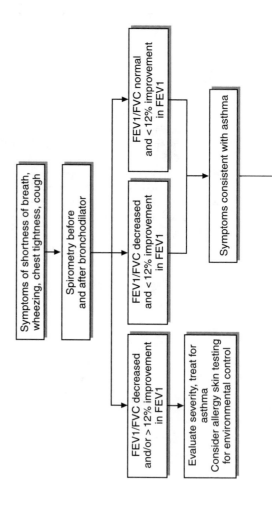

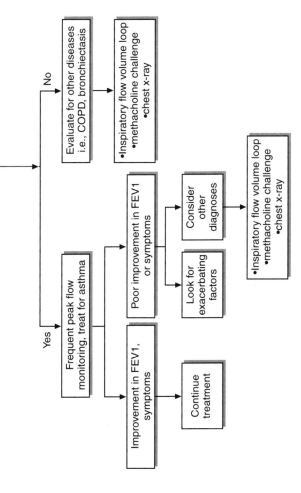

FIGURE 7.1. Strategy for the diagnosis and initial management of asthma.
EVIDENCE LEVEL: C. Expert Opinion.

STRATEGY FOR THE DIAGNOSIS AND INITIAL MANAGEMENT OF ASTHMA

135

TABLE 7.2. CLASSIFICATION OF ASTHMA SEVERITY

	Symptoms	Nighttime Symptoms	Lung Function
Step 1: mild, intermittent	Symptoms ≤2×/week; asymptomatic, normal peak flows between exacerbations; exacerbations brief (hours to days)	≤2×/month	FEV_1 or peak flow >80% predicted, peak flow variability <20%
Step 2: mild, persistent	Symptoms >2×/week, but <1×/day; exacerbations possibly affecting activity	>2×/month	FEV_1 or peak flow ≥80% predicted, peak flow variability 20–30%
Step 3: moderate, persistent	Daily symptoms, daily use of inhaled short-acting $β_2$-agonist, exacerbations affecting activity, exacerbations >2×/week	>1×/week	FEV_1 or peak flow between 60% and 80% predicted, peak flow variability >30%
Step 4: severe, persistent	Continual symptoms, limited physical activity, frequent exacerbations	Frequent	FEV_1 or peak flow <60% predicted, peak flow variability >30%

FEV_1, forced expiratory volume in 1 second.

EVIDENCE LEVEL: A. Reference: National Asthma Education and Prevention Program. Expert Panel Report II: Guidelines for the diagnosis and management of asthma. National Heart, Lung, and Blood Institute 1997;146.

TABLE 7.3. STEPWISE APPROACH FOR MANAGING ASTHMA IN ADULTS AND CHILDREN >5 YEARS OLD

	Long-Term Control	Quick Relief	Education
Step 1: mild, intermittent	None needed	Inhaled β-agonist for symptom relief	Basic asthma facts Basic inhaler/spacer techniques Discuss roles of medications Develop self-management plan Develop asthma action plan Discuss environmental control
Step 2: mild, persistent	One daily medication Anti-inflammatory: inhaled corticosteroid (low doses) Cromolyn/nedocromil Alternatively Theophylline Leukotriene modulator	Inhaled β-agonist for symptom relief	Step 1 actions plus Teach self-monitoring Refer to group education Review/update self-management plan
Step 3: moderate, persistent	Daily medications Anti-inflammatory: medium dose inhaled corticosteroid or Inhaled corticosteroid (low- to medium dose) with long-acting bronchodilator (long-acting β₂-agonist or theophylline If needed Medium to high dose of inhaled corticosteroids and long-acting bronchodilator (as above)	Inhaled β-agonist for symptom relief	As for step 2

| Step 4: severe, persistent | Daily medications
Anti-inflammatory
Inhaled corticosteroids (high dose) and long-acting
bronchodilator (long-acting β-agonist or
theophylline) and oral corticosteroids | Inhaled β-agonist
for symptom
relief | As for steps 1–3
Refer to individual education/
counseling |

EVIDENCE LEVEL: A. Reference: National Asthma Education and Prevention Program. Expert Panel Report II: Guidelines for the diagnosis and management of asthma. National Heart, Lung, and Blood Institute 1997;146.

STEPWISE APPROACH FOR MANAGING ASTHMA IN ADULTS AND CHILDREN

Algorithm for Acute Airway Compromise

upper airway distress

- air hunger
- stridor
- increased work of breathing
- costal retractions
- cyanosis
- tachypnea

Assess Pace and Degree of Obstruction

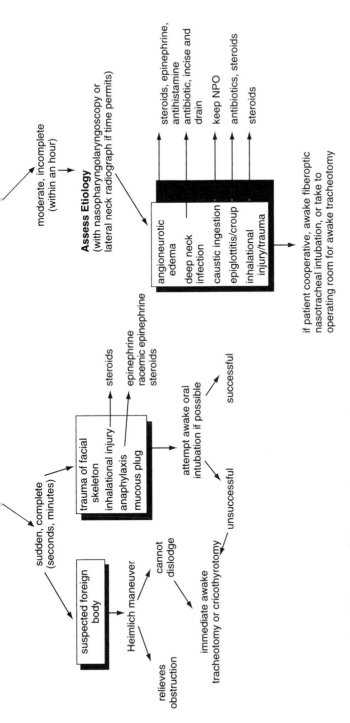

FIGURE 7.4. Algorithmic approach for acute airway compromise.
EVIDENCE LEVEL: C. Expert Opinion.

APPROACH FOR ACUTE AIRWAY COMPROMISE

141

TABLE 7.5.	INTERPRETATION OF SEVERITY OF RESTRICTIVE AND OBSTRUCTIVE LUNG DISEASE (BASED ON PHYSIOLOGIC MEASUREMENTS OF TLC AND FEV_1)	

Interpretation	TLC for Restriction (% of Predicted)	FEV_1 for Obstruction (% of Predicted)
Within normal limits	≥ 90	≥ 90
Within normal limits but is a low-normal: could also be mild restriction (obstruction)	80–90	LLN–90
Below limits of normal; most likely mild restriction (obstruction); small chance this is a variant of normal	70–80	70–LLN
Moderate restriction (obstruction)	60–70	60–70
Moderately severe restriction (obstruction)	50–60	50–60
Severe restriction (obstruction)	<50	<50

TLC, total lung capacity; FEV_1, forced expiratory volume in 1 second; LLN, lower limit of normal.

EVIDENCE LEVEL: B. Reference: American Thoracic Society Official Statement: Lung function testing: selection of reference values and interpretative strategies. *Am Rev Respir Dis* **1991;144:1202–1218.**

TABLE 7.6. A SCORING SYSTEM FOR PREDICTION OF MORTALITY

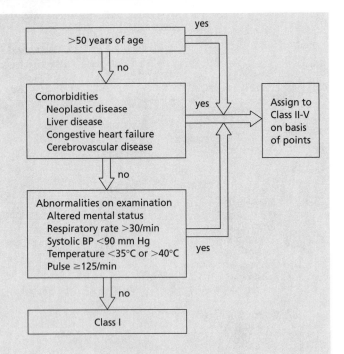

Category (points)	Mortality rate (%)
I (algorithm)	0.1–0.4
II (≤70)	0.6–0.7
III (71–90)	0.9–2.8
IV (91–130)	8.2–9.3
V (>130)	27–31

BP, blood pressure; Bun, blood urea nitrogen.
(From Fine MH, Auble TE, Yealy DM, et al. A predicton rule to identify low-risk patients with community acquired pneumonia. *N Engl J Med* 1997;336:243–250, with permission.)

Patients' characteristics, scoring system
  Demographic factors
    Male age (years)   —
    Female age (years)   −10   —
    Nursing home resident   +10   —
  Comorbid illnesses
    Neoplastic disease   +30   —
    Liver disease   +20   —
    Congestive heart failure   +10   —
    Cerebrovascular disease   +10   —
    Renal disease   +10   —
  Physical examination
    Altered mental status   +20   —
    Respiratory rate ≥30 breaths/min   +20   —
    Systolic BP <90 mm Hg   +20   —
    Temperature <35°C or ≥40°C   +15   —
    Pulse ≥125 beats/min   +10   —
  Laboratory findings
    pH <7.35   +30   —
    BUN >10.7   +20   —
    Sodium <130 mEq/L   +20   —
    Glucose >13.9 mmol/L   +10   —
    Hematocrit <30%   +10   —
    PaO_2 <60 mm Hg or O_2 saturation
      <90%   +10   —
    Pleural effusion   +10   —
  Total   —

EVIDENCE LEVEL: C. Reference: Fine MJ, Auble TE, Yealy DM, et al. A prediction rule to identify low-risk patients with community acquired pneumonia. *N Engl J Med* 1997;336:243–250.

| TABLE 7.7. | RECOMMENDED REGIMENS FOR TREATMENT OF LATENT TUBERCULOUS INFECTION IN ADULTS |

Drug	Frequency and Duration	Comments
Isoniazid	Daily or twice weekly[a] for 6–9 mo	Nine months is the preferred duration
Rifampin plus pyrazinamide	Daily or twice weekly[a] for 2 mo	Rifabutin may be substituted in patients receiving PIs or NNRTIs[b]
Rifampin	Daily for 4 mo	For persons who cannot tolerate pyrazinamide

[a] DOT must be used for twice-weekly regimens
[b] Rifabutin may be used with certain PIs or NNRTIs, dose adjustment of rifabutin and/or the PIs may be necessary.
DOT, directly observed therapy; PI, protease inhibitor; NNRTI, non-nucleoside reverse transcriptase inhibitor.

EVIDENCE LEVEL: A. Reference: American Thoracic Society. Targeted tuberculin testing and treatment of latent tuberculosis infection. *Am J Respir Crit Care Med* 2000; 161:S221–S247.

TABLE 7.8. GENERAL CATEGORIES OF SLEEP DISORDERS

Excessive Daytime Sleepiness (Hypersomnolence)	Inability to Sleep (Insomnia)	Unusual Events at Night (Parasomnia)
Sleep apnea	Acute	Sleep terrors
Narcolepsy	Psychological stress	Sleep walking or talking
Primary CNS hypersomnolence	Physical illness	REM behavior disorder
Inadequate sleep time	Time zone travel	Nocturnal seizures
Periodic limb movement disorder	Chronic	
Severe depression	Psychiatric disorder	
Drugs	Conditioned insomnia	
	Poor sleep hygiene	
	Circadian rhythm disorders	
	Pain or medical disorder	
	Restless leg syndrome	

REM, rapid eye movement.

EVIDENCE LEVEL: C. Expert Opinion.

8

ENDOCRINOLOGY, METABOLISM, AND GENETICS

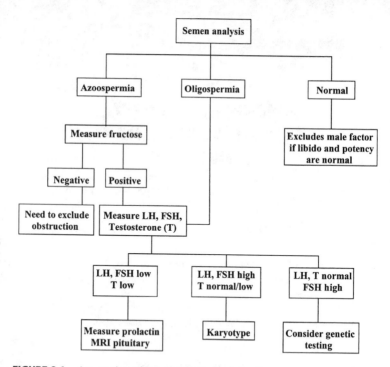

FIGURE 8.1. Approach to the evaluation of an infertile man.
EVIDENCE LEVEL: C. Expert Opinion.

TABLE 8.2.	**REPRESENTATIVE TARGET LEVELS FOR SELF-MONITORING OF BLOOD GLUCOSE LEVELS SUITABLE FOR A YOUNG, OTHERWISE HEALTHY PATIENT WITH TYPE I DIABETES IN A PROGRAM OF INTENSIVE THERAPY**		

Time	Ideal[a]	Acceptable[a]
Fasting/preprandial	70–105 mg/dL (3.9–5.8 mmol/L)	70–130 mg/dL (3.9–7.2 mmol/L)
Postprandial (1 hr)	100–160 mg/dL (5.6–8.9 mmol/L)	100–180 mg/dL (5.6–10.0 mmol/L)
Postprandial (2 hr)	80–120 mg/dL (4.4–6.7 mmol/L)	80–150 mg/dL (4.4–8.3 mmol/L)
Bedtime	100–140 mg/dL (5.6–7.8 mmol/L)	100–160 mg/dL (5.6–8.9 mmol/L)
2:00–4:00 a.m.	70–105 mg/dL (3.9–5.8 mmol/L)	70–130 mg/dL (3.9–7.2 mmol/L)

[a] Ideal values approximate those seen in nondiabetic individuals; they are included for illustrative purposes. Acceptable values are attainable in a reasonable number of patients without provoking undue hypoglycemia; they are provided to appropriate patients.

EVIDENCE LEVEL: C. Expert Opinion.

TABLE 8.3.   INDEXES OF GLYCEMIC CONTROL IN TYPE II DIABETES

Index	Ideal	Goal	Not Acceptable
Fasting/preprandial plasma glucose	<110 mg/dL (<6.1 mmol/L)	<120 mg/dL (<7.8 mmol/L)	<80 or >140 mg/dL (≥7.8 mmol/L)
Postprandial (2 hr) plasma glucose	<140 mg/dL (<7.8 mmol/L)	<180 mg/dL (<10.0 mmol/L)	>200 mg/dL (>11.1 mmol/L)
Bedtime plasma glucose	<140 mg/dL (<7.8 mmol/L)	100–140 mg/dL (5.6–8.9 mmol/L)	<100 or >160 mg/dL (<5.6 or >8.9 mmol/L)
Hb A$_{1c}$ (%)[a]	<6.0%	<7.0%	>8.0%
GHb (%)[b]	<7.0%	<8.0%	>9.5%

Hb A$_{1c}$, the major fraction of glycosylated hemoglobin.
[a] Referenced to a nondiabetic range of 4–6%.
[b] Referenced to a nondiabetic range of 4.5–7%.

EVIDENCE LEVEL: C. Expert Opinion.

TABLE 8.4. CHARACTERISTICS OF ORAL ANTIDIABETIC AGENTS AVAILABLE IN THE UNITED STATES

Generic Name	Brand Name	Dosage Range (mg/day)	Duration of Action (hr)	Dosing Frequency (per day)	Excretion
Sulfonylureas					
Tolbutamide	Orinase	500–3,000	6–12	2–3 times	Urine
Chlorpropamide	Diabinese	100–500	60	Once	Urine
Tolazamide	Tolinase	100–1,000	12–24	Twice	Urine
Acetohexamide	Dymelor	250–1,500	12–18	Twice	Urine
Glipizide	Glucotrol	2.5–40	12–24	Twice	Urine (Bile 20%)
Glipizide-GITS	Glucotrol XL	5–20	24	Once	Urine (bile 20%)
Glyburide	Diabeta micronase	1.25–20	16–24	Twice	Urine 50%, bile 50%
Glyburide (micronized)	Glynase	0.75–12	12–24	Twice	Urine 50%, bile 50%
Glimiperide	Amaryl	1–8	24	Once	Urine (bile 20%)
Miglitinides					
Repaglinide	Prandin	1.5–16	4–6	2–4 times ac	Bile
Nateglinide	Starlix	60–240	2–4	2–4 times ac	Urine
Biguanide					
Metformin	Glucophage	1,000–2,550	5–12	2–4 times	Urine
Thiazolidinediones					
Troglitazone	Rezulin	200–600	24	Once	Bile
Rosiglitazone	Avandia	4–8	15–25	1–2 times	Urine 70%, bile 30%
Pioglitazone	Actos	15–45	24–48	Once	Bile
α-Glucosidase inhibitor					
Acarbose	Precose	150–300	6	2–4 times ac	—
Miglitol	Glyset	75–600	6	2–4 times ac	—

TABLE 8.5. CAUSES OF HYPERTHYROIDISM

Graves' disease
Multinodular goiter
Hyperfunctioning thyroid adenoma (toxic adenoma)
Thyroiditis
  Subacute thyroiditis
  Painless (silent, postpartum) thyroiditis
Exogenous hyperthyroidism
  Thyroid hormone–induced hyperthyroidism
  Iodide-induced hyperthyroidism
Rare causes of hyperthyroidism
  TSH-secreting pituitary adenomas
  Trophoblastic tumors
  Struma ovarii
  Thyroid carcinoma
  Familial nonautoimmune hyperthyroidism

TSH, thyroid-stimulating hormone.
EVIDENCE LEVEL: C. Expert Opinion.

TABLE 8.6.	COMMON SYMPTOMS AND SIGNS OF HYPERTHYROIDISM

Symptoms

Anxiety, nervousness
Emotional lability
Easy fatigability
Increased perspiration
Heat intolerance
Palpitation
Dyspnea
Weakness
Weight loss
Increased appetite
Hyperdefecation

Signs

Hyperactivity
Eyelid retraction
Thyroid enlargement
Tachycardia (>90 beats/min)
Atrial fibrillation
Tremor
Muscle weakness
Hyperreflexia

EVIDENCE LEVEL: C. Expert Opinion.

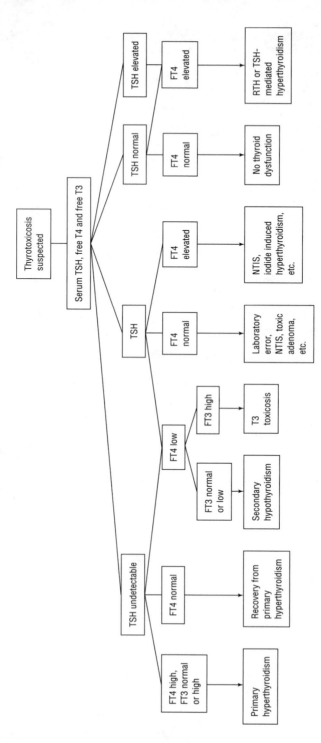

FIGURE 8.7. Strategies for Evaluation of Thyrotoxicosis. Evaluation should include careful history and physicial examination of the patient and should be individualized dependent on clinical situation. (TSH, thyroid-stimulating hormone, FT₃, free triiodothyronine; FT₄, free thyrozine, RTH, resistance to thyroid hormone, NTIS, non-thyroidal illness sysndrome).
EVIDENCE LEVEL: C. Expert Opinion.

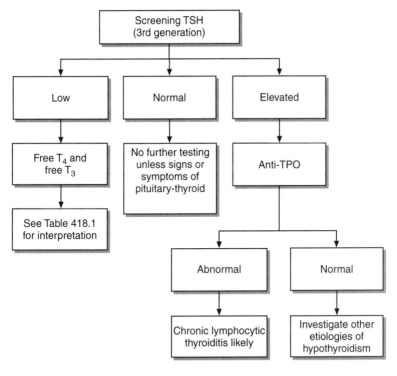

FIGURE 8.8. Thyroid function screening strategies based on serum TSH testing. **EVIDENCE LEVEL: C. Expert Opinion.**

TABLE 8.9. SYMPTOMS AND SIGNS OF HYPOTHYROIDISM

Symptoms

Weakness and fatigue
Lethargy
Decreased mental activity
Decreased physical activity
Dry skin
Decrease perspiration
Cold intolerance
Weight gain
Constipation
Paresthesia
Myalgia
Muscle and joint stiffness

Signs

Slow movements
Hoarse voice
Dry, cool skin
Periorbital edema
Edema of hands and feet
Goiter
Bradycardia
Slow relaxation of tendon reflexes

EVIDENCE LEVEL: C. Expert Opinion.

| TABLE 8.10. | CAUSES OF HYPOTHYROIDISM |

Primary (thyroidal) hypothyroidism
    Chronic autoimmune thyroiditis[a]
    ^{131}I or external-beam radiation therapy
    Postoperative hypothyroidism
    Transient hypothyroidism
    Infiltrative, diseases[a]
    Thyroid dysgenesis
    Defective thyroid hormone biosynthesis:
        Congenital defects[a]
        Iodide deficiency[a]
        Antithyroid agents[a]
        Iodine excess[a]
Secondary (central, hypothyrotropic) hypothyroidism
    Thyroid-stimulating hormone deficiency
    Thyrotropin-releasing hormone deficiency
Generalized resistance to thyroid hormone[a]

_____

[a] Goiter often present.
EVIDENCE LEVEL: C. Expert Opinion.

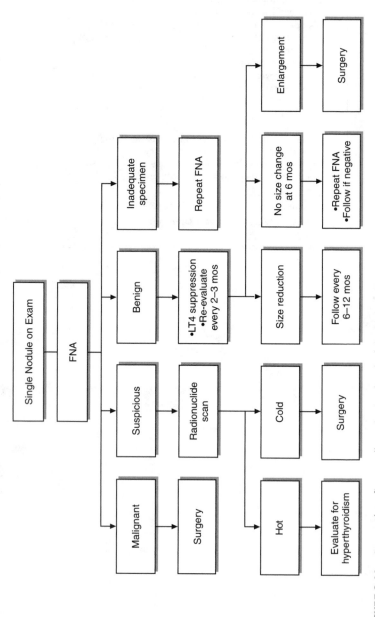

FIGURE 8.11. Approach to fine-needle aspiration (FNA) of single thyroid nodule.
EVIDENCE LEVEL: C. Expert Opinion.

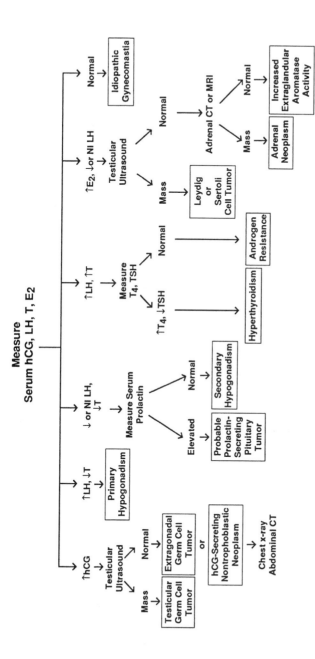

FIGURE 8.12. Evaluation of gynecomastia. hCG, human chorionic gonadotropin; LH, luteinizing hormone; T, testosterone; E_2, estradiol; T_4, thyroxine; TSH, thyroid-stimulating hormone; ↑, increased; ↓, decreased; Nl, normal. (From Braunstein GD. Gynecomastia. *N Engl J Med* 1993;328:490–495, with permission.)
EVIDENCE LEVEL: C. Expert Opinion.

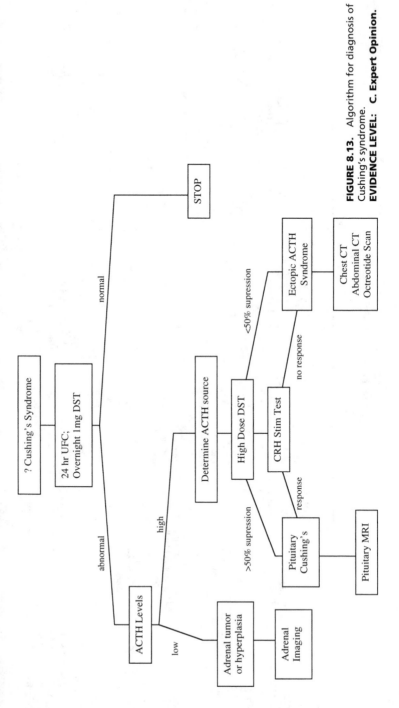

FIGURE 8.13. Algorithm for diagnosis of Cushing's syndrome. **EVIDENCE LEVEL: C. Expert Opinion.**

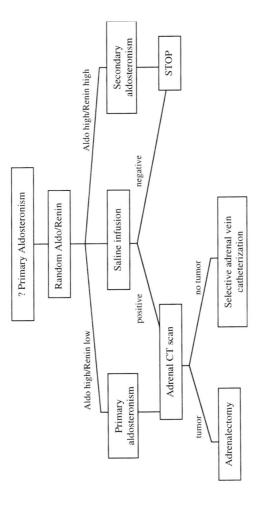

FIGURE 8.14. Diagnostic algorithm for patients suspected of having primary aldosteronism.
EVIDENCE LEVEL: C. Expert Opinion.

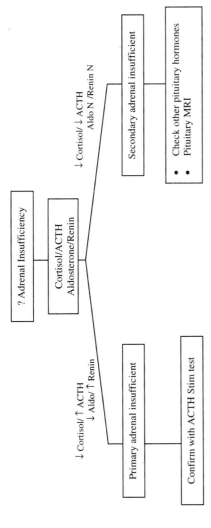

FIGURE 8.15. Diagnostic algorithm for patients suspected of having adrenal insufficiency.
EVIDENCE LEVEL: C. Expert Opinion.

PATIENTS SUSPECTED OF HAVING ADRENAL INSUFFICIENCY

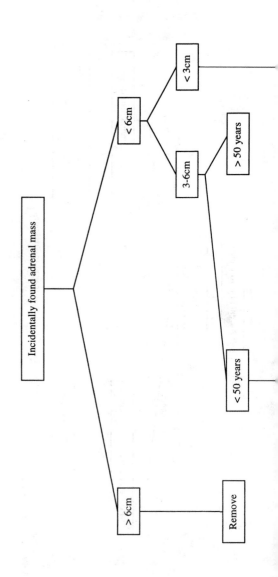

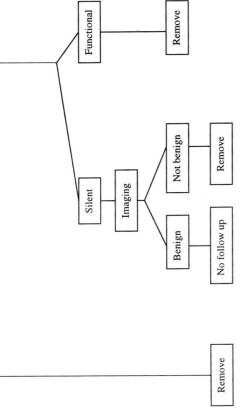

FIGURE 8.16. Algorithm for managing incidentally found adrenal masses.
EVIDENCE LEVEL: C. Expert Opinion.

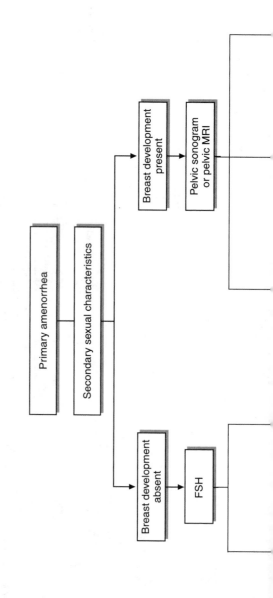

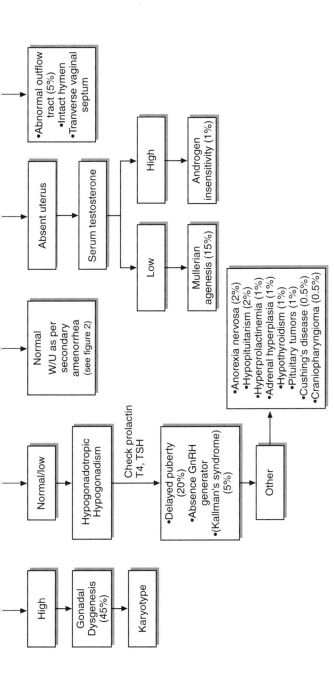

FIGURE 8.17. Causes of primary amenorrhea. FSH, follicle-stimulating hormone; GnRH, gonadotropin-releasing hormone; T₄, thyroxine; TSH, thyroid-stimulating hormone.
EVIDENCE LEVEL: C. Expert Opinion.

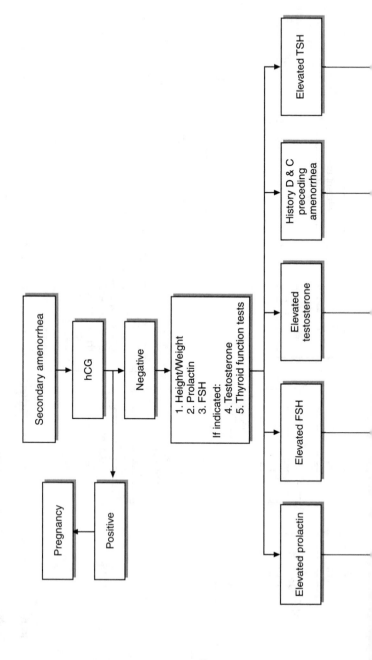

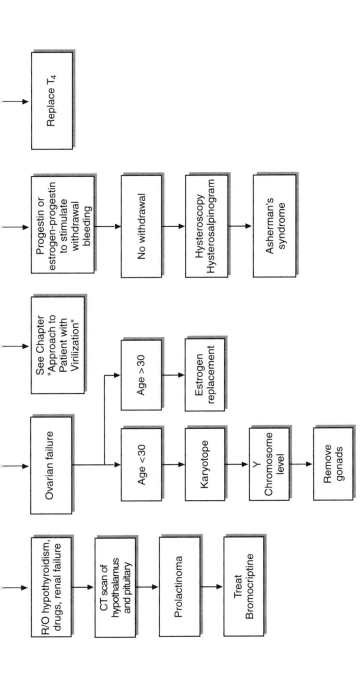

FIGURE 8.18. Major causes of secondary amenorrhea. CT, computed tomography; D&C, dilation and curettage; FSH, follicle-stimulating hormone; hCG, human chorionic gonadotropin; R/O, rule out; T₄, thyroxine. **EVIDENCE LEVEL: C. Expert Opinion.**

MAJOR CAUSES OF SECONDARY AMENORRHEA

9

NEUROLOGY

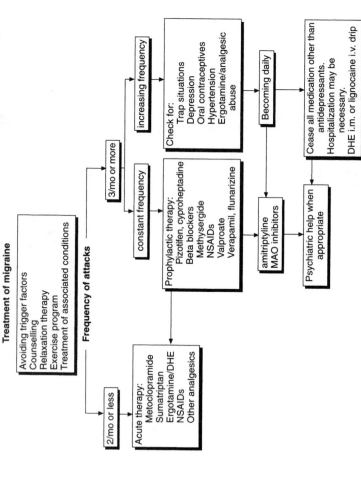

FIGURE 9.1. A logical sequence of therapy in the management of migraine headaches. DHE, dihydroergotamine; NSAIDs, nonsteroidal antiinflammatory drugs; MAO, monoamine oxidase. (Updated from a diagram first published in Current Therapeutics, April 1980. Reproduced by permission of Adis International 1994.)

**EVIDENCE LEVEL: B. Reference: Lance JW, Goadsby PJ. *Mechanisms and management of headache*, sixth edition. Butterworth-Heine-

TABLE 9.2. CEREBROSPINAL FLUID (CSF) FINDINGS IN BACTERIAL AND NONBACTERIAL MENINGITIS

CSF Profile	Bacterial	Viral	Mycobacterial or Fungal
Total cells (per µL)	Usually >500	Usually <500	Usually <500
White blood cells	Predominantly polymorphonuclear	Predominantly mononuclear	Predominantly mononuclear
Glucose (% of blood)	≤40%	>40%	≤40%
Protein (mg/dL)	>50	>50	>50
Gram stain	Positive (65–95%)	Negative	Negative

Differential diagnosis of CSF pleocytosis

Brain abscess or subdural empyema with rupture

Central nervous system vasculitis, tumor

Predominantly Polymorphonuclear (>90% PMNs)

Bacterial meningitis

Early viral meningitis

Early tuberculous or fungal meningitis

Brain abscess or subdural empyema with rupture into subarachnoid space

Chemical arachnoiditis

Brain abscess of subdural empyema

Predominantly Mononuclear (<90% PMNs)

Viral meningitis or encephalitis

Tuberculous or fungal meningitis

Partially treated bacterial meningitis

Brain abscess of subdural empyema

Listeriosis (variable)

Neurosyphilis

Neuroborreliosis (Lyme disease)

Neurocysticercosis

Primary amoebic meningoencephalitis

Guillain–Barre syndrome

Central nervous system vasculitis, tumor, hemorrhage

Multiple sclerosis

PMNs, polymorphonuclear leukocytes.

EVIDENCE LEVEL: B. Reference: Lepow ML, et al. Aseptic meningitis: clinical epidemiologic, and laboratory investigation during the four year period 1955–1958. *New Engl J Med* 1962;266:1181–1193.

TABLE 9.3. INITIAL EMPIRIC ANTIMICROBIAL THERAPY FOR ACUTE PURULENT MENINGITIS[a]

Age	Common Organisms	Recommended Therapy
0–4 wk	Escherichia coli, Streptococcus agalactiae, Listeria monocytogenes	Ampicillin plus third-generation cephalosporin[b] or ampicillin plus aminoglycoside
4–12 wk	E. coli, S. agalactiae, L. monocytogenes, Haemophilus influenzae, Streptococcus pneumoniae	Ampicillin plus third-generation cephalosporin[b]
3 mo to 18 yr	Neisseria meningitidis, S. pneumoniae, H. influenzae	Third-generation cephalosporin or ampicillin plus chloramphenicol
18–50 yr	S. pneumoniae, N. meningitidis	Third-generation cephalosporin[a] ± ampicillin
>50 yr	S. pneumoniae, N. meningitidis, L. monocytogenes, gram-negative bacilli	Ampicillin plus third-generation cephalosporin[b]

[a] Patients without underlying illness.
[b] Cefotaxime, ceftriaxone—vancomycin should be added if penicillin or cephalosporin-resistant *S. pneumoniae* is suspected.

EVIDENCE LEVEL: A. Reference: Tunkel AR, Wispelweg B, Scheld WM. Bacterial meningitis: recent advances in pathophysiology and treatment. Ann Intern Med 1990;122:610.

TABLE 9.4. RECOMMENDED DOSES OF ANTIBIOTICS FOR SUPPURATIVE INTRACRANIAL INFECTIONS IN ADULTS

Antibiotic	Daily	Dosing Interval (h)
Penicillin G	20–24 million units	4
Ampicillin	12 g	4
Nafcillin, oxacillin	9–12 g	4
Piperacillin	8–12 g	4
Imipenem	4–6 g	6
Cefotaxime	8–12 g	4
Ceftriaxone	4–6 g	12
Ceftizoxime	4–6 g	8
Ceftazidime	6–12 g	8
Chloramphenicol	4–6 g	6
Vancomycin	2 g	12
Gentamicin, tobramycin	3–5 mg/kg	8
Amikacin	15 mg/kg	8
Ciprofloxacin	200–400 mg	12
Metronidazole	30–60 mg/kg	6
Trimethoprim-sulfamethoxazole	5–10 mg/kg 25–50 mg/kg	12 12

EVIDENCE LEVEL: C. Reference: Expert Opinion.

TABLE 9.5.	PHYSICAL DIAGNOSIS OF COMA: RULES AND EXCEPTIONS

Symmetrical Signs, Brain Stem Functions Intact

Rule: Cause of coma most likely is metabolic or diffuse. Concentrate on metabolic, toxic, and infectious sources.

Exception: Early central herniation (see text) due to a supratentorial mass lesion may mimic metabolic encephalopathy.

Asymmetrical Signs, Brain Stem Functions Intact

Rule: Cause of coma is probably an acute hemisphere mass lesion. Treat urgently to check further herniation.

Exception: Hypoglycemic and hepatic encephalopathy may produce asymmetrical signs, but usually asymmetries do not persist. Metabolic encephalopathy superimposed on a previous neurological deficit may cause confusion in diagnosis.

Symetrical Signs, Caudal Brain Stem Functions Impaired

Rule: Cause of coma is most likely intoxication or metabolic encephalopathy.

Exception: A posterior fossa mass lesion causing rostral to caudal deterioration may mimic metabolic coma.

Asymmetrical Signs of Brain Stem Dysfunction

Rule: Cause of coma is most likely a structural lesion of the posterior fossa. Consider basilar artery thrombosis, pontine hemorrhage, and cerebellar infarct or hematoma.

Exception: None

EVIDENCE LEVEL: B. Reference: Stuben JP, Caronna JJ. Coma. In: Parillo JE, ed. *Current therapy in critical care medicine,* third edition. St. Louis: Mosby, 1977:306–310.

TABLE 9.6. GLASGOW COMA SCALE[a]

Parameter	Score
Eye opening	
Spontaneous	4
To speech	3
To noxious stimulation	2
None	1
Best Motor Response	
Obeys commands	6
Localizes stimuli	5
Withdraws	4
Abnormal flexion	3
Extensor response	2
None	1
Verbal Response	
Oriented	5
Confused conversation	4
Inappropriate words	3
Incomprehensible sounds	2
None	1

[a] The coma score is the sum of individual scores for eye opening, motor, and verbal response of 3–15.

EVIDENCE LEVEL: A. Reference: Teasdale G, Jennett B. Assessment of coma and impaired consciousness: a practical scale. *Lancet* **1974;2:81.**

TABLE 9.7. CRITERIA FOR PANIC ATTACK[a]

A discrete period of intense fear or discomfort in which at least four of the following symptoms develop abruptly.
Chest pain or discomfort
Palpitations, cardiac awareness, or accelerated heart rate
Sweating
Trembling or shaking
Sensation of shortness of breath or smothering
Feeling of choking
Nausea or abdominal distress
Feeling dizzy, unsteady, lightheaded, or faint
Feelings of unreality or detachment from oneself
Fear of losing control or going crazy
Fear of dying
Numbness or tingling sensations
Chills or hot flashes

---

[a] Diagnostic and Statistical Manual for Mental Disorders (DSM-IV).

EVIDENCE LEVEL: B. Reference: American Psychiatric Association. *Diagnostic and statistical manual of mental disorders, fourth edition.* **Washington, DC: American Psychiatric Association, 1994.**

10

GERIATRICS

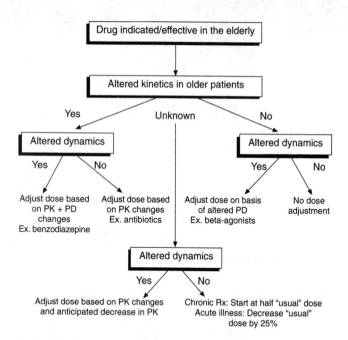

FIGURE 10.1. Schematic representation of the steps involved in choosing a therapeutic dosage regimen for an older patient.
EVIDENCE LEVEL: C. Expert Opinion.

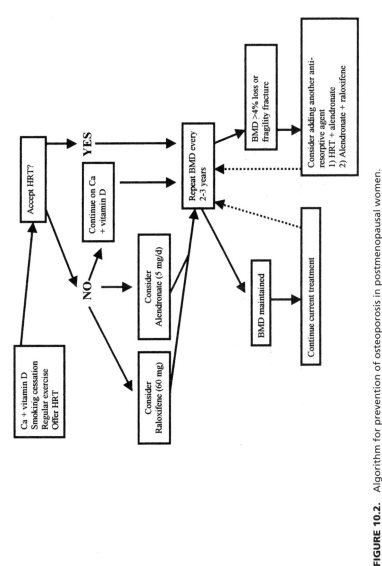

FIGURE 10.2. Algorithm for prevention of osteoporosis in postmenopausal women.
EVIDENCE LEVEL: B. Reference: National Osteoporosis Foundation. Physicians guide to prevention and treatment of osteoporosis.
Belle Meade, NJ: Excerpta Medica, 1998.

THERAPEUTIC DOSING REGIMEN FOR AN OLDER PATIENT

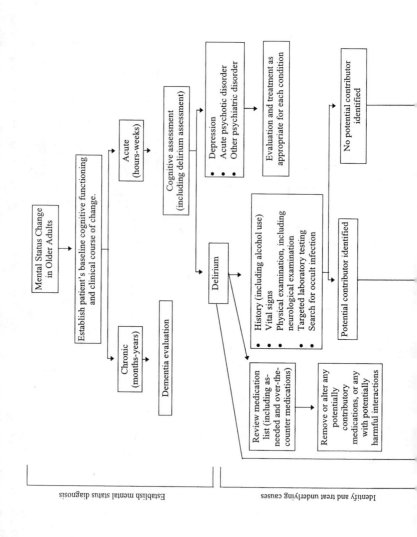

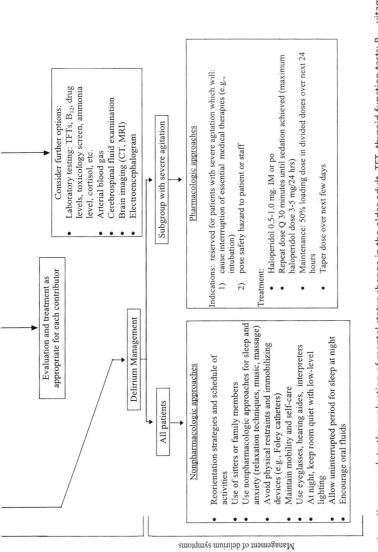

FIGURE 10.3. A systematic approach to the evaluation of mental status change in the older adult. TFT, thyroid function tests; B_{12}, vitamin B_{12} assay; CT, computed tomography; MRI, magnetic resonance imaging; IM, intramuscular injection; PO, oral administration.
EVIDENCE LEVEL: C. Expert Opinion.

185

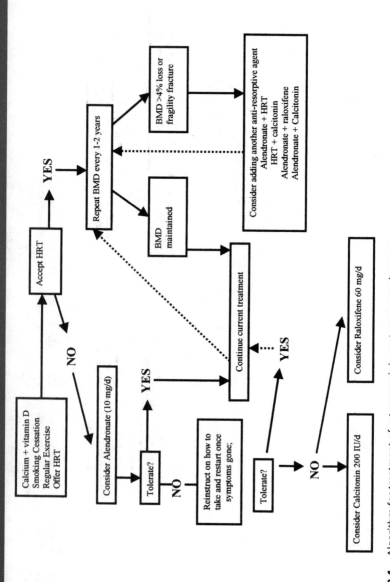

FIGURE 10.4. Algorithm for treatment of osteoporosis in postmenopausal women.
EVIDENCE LEVEL: B. Reference: National Osteoporosis Foundation. Physicians guide to prevention and treatment of osteoporosis. Belle Meade, NJ: Excerpta Medica, 1998.

Index of Clinical Decision Guides

Page numbers for figures also found in the fourth edition of *Kelley's Textbook of Internal Medicine,* are provided in italic.